First World War Nursing

This book brings together a collection of works by scholars who have produced some of the most innovative and influential work on the topic of First World War nursing in the last ten years. The contributors employ an interdisciplinary collaborative approach that takes into account multiple facets of Allied wartime nursing: historical contexts (history of the profession, recruitment, teaching, different national socio-political contexts), popular cultural stereotypes (in propaganda, popular culture) and longstanding gender norms (woman-as-nurturer). They draw on a wide range of hitherto neglected historical sources, including diaries, novels, letters and material culture. The result is a fully-rounded new study of nurses' unique and compelling perspectives on the unprecedented experiences of the First World War.

Alison S. Fell is Professor of French Cultural History at the University of Leeds.

Christine E. Hallett is Professor of Nursing History at the University of Manchester, UK.

Routledge Studies in Modern History

1 **Isolation**
Places and Practices of Exclusion
Edited by Carolyn Strange and Alison Bashford

2 **From Slave Trade to Empire**
European Colonisation of Black Africa 1780s–1880s
Edited by Olivier Pétré Grenouilleau

3 **Revolution, Counter-Revolution and Revisionism in Postcolonial Africa**
The Case of Mozambique, 1975–1994
Alice Dinerman

4 **Charity and Mutual Aid in Europe and North America since 1800**
Edited by Paul Bridgen and Bernard Harris

5 **Churchill, Roosevelt and India**
Propaganda During World War II
Auriol Weigold

6 **Genocide and Fascism**
The Eliminationist Drive in Fascist Europe
Aristotle Kallis

7 **Scientific Research in World War II**
What Scientists Did in the War
Edited by Ad Maas and Hans Hooijmaijers

8 **Restoration and History**
The Search for a Useable Environmental Past
Edited by Marcus Hall

9 **Foundations of Modernity**
Human Agency and the Imperial State
Isa Blumi

10 **Transpacific Revolutionaries**
The Chinese Revolution in Latin America
Matthew D. Rothwell

11 **First World War Nursing**
New Perspectives
Edited by Alison S. Fell and Christine E. Hallett

First World War Nursing

New Perspectives

**Edited by Alison S. Fell
and Christine E. Hallett**

Routledge
Taylor & Francis Group
NEW YORK LONDON

First published 2013
by Routledge
711 Third Avenue, New York, NY 10017

Simultaneously published in the UK
by Routledge
2 Park Square, Milton Park, Abingdon, Oxon OX14 4RN

Routledge is an imprint of the Taylor & Francis Group,
an informa business

Library of Congress Cataloging-in-Publication Data

First World War nursing : new perspectives / edited by Alison S. Fell and
Christine E. Hallett.
pages cm. — (Routledge studies in modern history ; 11)
Includes bibliographical references and index.
1. World War, 1914–1918—Medical care. 2. World War, 1914–1918—Medical care—Sources. 3. Military nursing—History—20th century. 4. Military nursing—History—20th century—Sources. 5. Nurses—History—20th century. 6. Nurses—History—20th century—Sources. 7. World War, 1914–1918—Participation, Female. 8. World War, 1914–1918—Participation, Female—Sources. I. Fell, Alison S., 1971– II. Hallett, Christine E.
D628.F57 2013
940.4'75—dc23
2012047862

ISBN13: 978-0-415-83205-2 (hbk)
ISBN13: 978-0-203-44892-2 (ebk)

Typeset in Sabon
by IBT Global.

Contents

Figures

Acknowledgments

The editors would like to thank the Wellcome Trust for their support of the workshop in which the contributors to this volume were able to discuss their contributions and share their insights. We would also like to express our gratitude to the anonymous readers for their helpful comments and advice, and the contributors for their scholarly engagement and enthusiasm. Extracts from Mary Brown's diary are reproduced by kind permission of Mrs. E. Cleverly OBE; quotations from Vera Brittain are included by permission of Mark Bostridge and T. J. Brittain-Catlin, Literary Executors for the Estate of Vera Brittain 1970; the quotation from Mary Knocker's unpublished memoir *Through Shadows and Sunshine, 1914–1918*, is included by permission of the Wellcome Library (from the Papers of Mary Ethel Corry Knocker [later Love] [1883–1970]); Mary Borden's unpublished poem is reproduced by permission of Duff Hart-Davis; and quotations from Alice Alment née Slythe are included by permission of Mrs. Molly Currie. Every effort has been made to contact the copyright holders of the following two texts: Enid Bagnold, *A Diary Without Dates*; Irene Rathbone, *We That Were Young. A Novel.* The editors acknowledge the valuable contribution of these two texts to Chapter Five of this book.

Introduction
New Perspectives on First World War Nursing

Christine E. Hallett and Alison S. Fell

Anyone reading the histories of the First World War produced in the five decades that followed it could have been forgiven for assuming that participation in the conflict was an exclusively masculine experience. A pivotal moment in this trend was the publication in the 1970s of Paul Fussell's *The Great War and Modern Memory*,[1] which is widely viewed as representing the apotheosis of this male-dominated perspective, yet which simultaneously opened the way for a new genre of writing about the First World War as a culturally transformative event.[2] Responding to both the challenge and the prompt posed by Fussell's work, women's historians have, from the 1970s onward, worked to rectify the imbalance within the historical record: to restore women to their place in the history of the First World War. Their works collectively introduced new sources, as well as contributing to an innovative gendered understanding of war and its consequences. In a search for women who can be understood as active participants rather than passive observers of war, many historians and cultural critics began to research and consider the role, image, and experiences of First World War nurses.[3]

The chapters in this volume focus on the thousands of women from the Allied nations who worked as nurses during the First World War. In Britain the military medical authorities had a small but well-established military nursing service on which to draw (in addition to the thousands of trained nurses who worked in civilian hospitals). The British military nursing services consisted of: the Queen Alexandra's Imperial Military Nursing Service (QAIMNS), the Queen Alexandra's Imperial Military Nursing Service Reserve (QAIMNSR), and the Territorial Force Nursing Service (TFNS).[4] These military nurses, who numbered around twenty-three hundred in the early months of the war,[5] were aided by the Voluntary Aid Detachments (VAD), which had been formed in 1909 to assist the work of the QAIMNS and the TFNS and were organized under the auspices of the British Red Cross Society and the Order of Saint John of Jerusalem. On the outbreak of war thousands more volunteered, and the end of the war over seventy thousand women had served as VADs.[6] British numbers of nurses were also swelled from 1915 onward by the arrival of trained military nurses from Canada, Australia, New Zealand, and South Africa, who worked in all theaters. In addition, there were British professional and volunteer nurses attached to organizations such as the Belgian and French Red Cross, the French Flag Nursing Corps, the Scottish Women's Hospitals, and the Women's Sick and Wounded Convoy Corps, or to one of the privately funded initiatives such as the hospitals set up in France by the Duchess of Sutherland and Duchess of Westminster. These organizations also recruited American volunteers, many of them wealthy women who could afford to travel and support their hospital work from their private incomes. Other American women, such as Mary Borden, set up their own hospitals under the auspices of the French military medical services.[7] Subsequently, when the US entered the war in 1917, further trained military nurses were mobilized. Over twenty-one thousand women served in the US Army Nurse Corps, 10,660 of them with the American Expeditionary Force.[8]

France also supplied large numbers of nurses, including about six thousand professional nurses employed by the French state authorities (the *Assistance publique*), and others attached to military hospitals.[9] By far the largest percentage of French First World War nurses, totaling more than one hundred thousand by the end of 1918, worked as nurses for one of the three organizations that made up the French Red Cross, of which about thirty thousand were paid.[10] In addition, there were approximately ten thousand women from religious orders who worked in wartime hospitals.[11] In Russia, the numbers of Red Cross nurses, who were recruited from "Sisters of Mercy" communities that were founded by aristocratic women in the nineteenth century, were relatively low at the outbreak of war, at about four thousand.[12] Training courses were shortened in a bid to recruit more women, and by 1916 their ranks had swelled to twenty-five thousand, although there remained a serious shortage of qualified Russian medical personnel throughout the war.[13] Other Allied nations, in which both military nursing and nursing as a profession were still in their infancy in comparison to Britain and the US, equally struggled to provide significant numbers of trained nurses at the outbreak of the war. As in Russia, Italian nurses were drawn from the volunteer sector, and only around eight thousand nurses worked for the Italian Red Cross during the war.[14]

Romania and Serbia also recruited volunteer nurses for their respective Red Cross Societies, which had been training volunteers and raising funds since the First Balkan War. These volunteers were often from the upper echelons of society, and as in other nations included members of royal families such as Queen Marie of Romania, who carried out fundraising activities and helped to raise the profile of the Red Cross.[15] But such efforts proved inadequate as the situation in Serbia and Romania was particularly acute in 1915 and 1916, with cholera and typhus epidemics adding to the obstacles already caused by the disadvantages of operating in an occupied country. It is estimated that 65 percent of Serbia's military deaths were due to disease rather than enemy action, and a severe shortage of trained personnel, both doctors and nurses, led to calls for help from the Allied nations via the International Red Cross Society.[16] This was quickly forthcoming; organizations from Russia and Britain had already sent teams of doctors and nurses during the Balkan Wars. Many of the surviving sources describing conditions and experiences in hospitals at the Serbian front, such as those discussed in Angela Smith's chapter, are therefore from the perspective of British women who volunteered to go there with organizations like the Serbian Relief Fund.[17] Belgium, like Serbia, was a nation that welcomed nurses from a range of Allied organizations as it had relatively few trained nurses at the outbreak of the war. For example, Dr. Antoine Depage, Belgian doctor and president of its Red Cross Society, recruited several British and French nurses for his well-known Hôtel de l'Océan hospital at La Panne.[18] In some cases, the International Red Cross facilitated this movement of medical personnel from one Allied nation to another. Small teams of Red Cross nurses were sent, for instance, to Russia, France, and Britain from Japan and Norway. The arrival of the Japanese nurses in particular was widely covered by the press.[19] In other cases, individuals or smaller national organizations carried out fundraising and made their own arrangements. Thus, although some trained women, such as British female doctors, were frustrated by the unwillingness of their national authorities to use their skills, "so urgent was the Allies' need for medical care" in certain theaters that "a woman could find work on her own initiative."[20]

In some of the first published studies of First World War nursing, all women who worked in some capacity in wartime hospitals were considered to be "nurses"—mirroring, in effect, First World War popular understandings of nursing as women's "natural" and most vital role in wartime, an extension of their domestic roles as carers and nurturers. However, it remains important for several reasons to distinguish between trained nurses and volunteers. As Janet Watson's chapter demonstrates, the perspective of an experienced professional who had already witnessed medical trauma was bound to differ from that of an inexperienced volunteer, and it is important to identify and explore these differences.[21] In the eyes of the general public, volunteer nurses were more prominent than their professional colleagues, to whom they owed much of their training and support. This is most obviously the case within the British context, where the VAD nurse had a higher public profile—both during the war and since—than the trained professional nurses of both the QAIMNS and the TFNS, and this sometimes caused tension and mutual resentment between individuals, as Christine Hallett notes in her chapter.[22] But similar rivalries existed in France: Yvonne Knibiehler and Katrin Schultheiss outline not only the fierce competition that existed between the three different French Red Cross organizations, but equally the extent to which the rise of the volunteer nurse, understood as an extension of womanhood itself in the public imagination, proved an obstacle to the trained *Assistance Publique* and military nurses who were engaged in a struggle for higher pay and greater professionalization.[23]

Modern scholarship within the emerging field of nursing history is working to rectify the focus on volunteer rather than professional nurses by some historians, just as the earliest women's historians worked to restore the gender imbalance they encountered in male-focused histories of the conflict.[24] Intersecting with women's studies and also with the fields of medical history and military history, the history of nursing is beginning to both develop its own perspective and engage with those of other disciplines. This volume seeks to continue this development, by deploying through its contributions an interdisciplinary, collaborative approach to the study of First World War nursing that seeks to unearth new perspectives and insights. By taking into account multiple facets of wartime nursing—historical contexts, popular cultural stereotypes, variation in individual experience (between trained and volunteer nurses, between belligerent nations, and between different theaters of war)—it aims to produce a fully rounded analysis of the sources, and in particular of the complex narrative layers of the autobiographical texts—the novels, memoirs, letters, and diaries—produced by nurses during and after the war. The contributions explore, firstly, the First World War nurse as cultural construct, assessing the extent to which images of nursing draw on pre-existing stereotypes, or develop new idealized models of female identity as a result of the exceptional circumstances brought about by the war and its aftermath. Secondly, they consider both professional and volunteer nurses as historical actors, exploring in particular the ways in which they recorded their experiences in their writings.

The first part of the volume considers the relationship of nurses to the national identities forged in war, taking as case studies France, Britain, and America. Although the prominence in all Allied nations of the wartime nurse as a national heroine is generally understood to be a feature of the First World War, Margaret Darrow traces its origins and development in France back to the nineteenth century. Her chapter reveals that the qualities of courage, martial spirit, and religious devotion that characterize First World War French nursing heroines such as Sister Julie, who achieved national renown, were already present in the myths and narratives of the Franco-Prussian War and the interwar period. She demonstrates that the development of a collection of popular myths expounding the heroism of female nurses fed the enthusiasm with which untrained women flocked to offer their services to the French military medical services at the outbreak of war. Among those who had been lauded for their contribution to the earlier conflict were nuns, aristocratic ladies, and famous actresses who had established makeshift ambulances in venues ranging from chateaux—which were often easily adapted to create hospital wards—to highly unsuitable premises such as the foyers of theaters. At the outbreak of the First World War, the request of the French authorities that offers of nursing service should only be made by those who were suitably qualified fell largely on deaf ears, as women of all backgrounds (but particularly members of the social elite) keen to contribute to the war effort drew on this rich fund of mythology about the capacity of French women to offer devoted service to their own wounded, whether trained or not.

Angela Smith's chapter considers the importance of a sense of "Britishness" for nurses and female doctors who remained "at their posts" in hospital units in Serbia during the German/Bulgarian invasion of 1915. Drawing on several evocative diaries, she addresses the ways in which these women expressed a patriotic sense of themselves as Britons in the face of the oppression of their captors, the reproaches of the Serbian people, and the apparent indifference of their own government. Smith offers a clear impression of the Serbian front as forgotten or invisible—the lowest priority for the Allied armies who, in 1915, were heavily preoccupied with the deadlock on the western front and the failure to break through on the Gallipoli peninsula. Yet women such as Leila Paget, Elsie Inglis, and Alice Hutchison chose to stay as prisoners of war in Serbia rather than return to Britain. The chapter suggests that a deeply embedded sense of imperialism enabled these women to see themselves as "beacons of Britishness" who had a duty to stay in a foreign land and represent the values of the empire—although such a position was inevitably complicated by the fact that, as carers, their duty was to prioritize their sick and wounded, embodying an ideal of transnational humanitarianism.

An analysis of lesser-known writings of women who traveled to different fronts during the First World War can, in this way, offer insights into the ways in which those who worked as nurses—both professional and volunteer—experienced the moral and emotional challenges of engagement in warfare. Jane Potter's chapter considers the way in which many of the American women who volunteered in European hospitals during the war positioned themselves in moral terms in relation, first, to their nation's neutrality and, second, to its entry in the war. She therefore uses the published writings of these women—now largely forgotten—as a lens through which we can view the complexities of the American response to war. From the early years of the conflict in which a few enthusiasts, many of whom were viewed as "dilettantes" and "war-tourists," offered their services to institutions such as the American Ambulance in Paris, to the months following April 1917 in which the American nation threw itself wholesale into the conflict, these writings mirror the complexities of the American emotional response to the war. From "detached spectator" to "crusading participant," the majority of accounts of the war published by American authors appear to have been infused by a naïve assurance that the role of the US in world affairs was to make the world "safe for democracy"—although, as Potter remarks, it should be borne in mind that the publication of these texts was often motivated by a desire to promote and justify America's joining of the Allied cause. However, in the later years of the war, and as the real horror of its consequences became apparent, these American nurse-writers began to express the ethical "double bind" that was experienced by those who believed that their role was to engage heroically in a just cause and yet found themselves acting as participants in a war of apparently meaningless destruction. Their powerful writings bear witness to their hesitations and moral uncertainties in relation to this dilemma.

The second part of the volume focuses on professional nurses, whose skills, perspectives, and sense of their own identities evolved as they experienced the unprecedented conditions of First World War hospitals and dressing stations. In her contribution, Kirsty Harris focuses on the nurturing aspects of the professional nursing work carried out by Australian military nurses, arguing that war not only transformed their nursing practice, but also changed nurse–patient relationships, especially in the context of Australian women nursing their fellow countrymen. She draws on a range of nurses' letters and diaries in order to identify five key components—trust, respect, professional intimacy, empathy, and power—that structured these relationships. She emphasizes in particular the tendency of many nurses to stretch or break professional boundaries in wartime and take a personal interest in their patients' well-being. One of the most interesting features of wartime nursing—and one found quite frequently in nurses' own writings—was the tendency to deliberately take on nurturing roles that mirrored those of absent family caregivers: mothers and sisters. This theme finds particular emphasis in the writings of these Australian Army Nursing Service sisters, whose diaries, letters, and narratives often refer to the closeness and camaraderie of their relationships with their patients.

Although Harris notes the extent to which nurse–patient relationships shifted and evolved during the war, one of the features of military nursing in the first decades of the twentieth century remained the capacity of nurses for placing firm boundaries between the personal and professional. This could sometimes have the consequence—disconcerting for the historian—that personal letters and diaries have a superficial feel and contain a frustrating lack of evidence of the actual work performed by nurses.[25] Christine Hallett's *Containing Trauma* (2009) has demonstrated that a careful search for more informative material can yield results.[26] Nevertheless, it remains the case that for every brief account of a professional nurse's work there can be found many pages of material relating to her travel, her living conditions, and the foibles of her colleagues. These findings are undoubtedly, in large part, a consequence of censorship, both by the state and by the nurse herself. Self-censorship was a complex phenomenon. A nurse might withhold material for a number of reasons, ranging from a desire to protect her relatives from the sordid truth to a careful attention to what might or might not safely pass the official censor's gaze.[27] Yet the absence of this material may also be a consequence of deliberate emotional distancing. The emotional content of the military nurse's work is examined in Hallett's chapter through the published writings of both professional and volunteer nurses. The military hospital ward was a highly charged environment. Wounded men often experienced an emotional trajectory from fear and despair on first arriving at a base hospital to relief and even elation as they moved from an acute to a convalescent state, followed by boredom at the constraints of hospital military discipline. Their behavior could mirror this emotional trajectory, ranging from acute distress, occasional confusion, and angry outbursts to enthusiastic engagement in their own rehabilitation, boisterousness, and deliberate attempts to subvert hospital discipline. The boredom of hospital routine, punctuated only by meals, washes, and the daily dressing round led these young, healthy recovering patients to find an outlet for their emotions by engaging in banter and horseplay. Some volunteer nurses saw no problem in participating in such "high jinks," as the writings of individuals such as Vera Brittain and Irene Rathbone illustrate.[28] By contrast, professional nurses had been trained to maintain a safe emotional distance between themselves and their patients, and they had an acute awareness of what they saw as the potential dangers of emotional entanglement. VADs, without such training and experience, were more inclined to engage with their patients in what they saw as a natural and friendly manner. These relationships were sometimes further complicated by differences of social class and background between patients and nurses.

Drawing on the writings of both trained and volunteer nurses, Hallett shows that these distinctions in manner and behavior were interpreted in different ways by the two groups. VADs saw nurses as overly detached and impersonal, while nurses saw VADs as excessively involved with their patients, often in a way that aroused suspicion that a volunteer's motives in entering the hospital environment had more to do with a search for romance and adventure than a desire to do nursing work. She concludes that professional nurses' and VADs' critiques of each other's behavior may have had their origins more in their behavior toward each other than in their actual attitudes to patients. Of real significance to well-known VAD writers such as Brittain, Rathbone, and Enid Bagnold was the bullying behavior of some trained nurses. In Rathbone's case, this was most particularly the matron of the First London General Hospital, Rachael Cox-Davies, whose behavior she parodied as being that of an unthinking martinet,[29] while in *Diary without Dates* Enid Bagnold presented an even more devastating expose of the behavior of nurses at the Royal Herbert Hospital in Woolwich, which she depicted as thoughtless and callous.[30]

The tendency for some professional nurses to distance themselves from the emotional content of their work is amply illustrated by Janet Watson's chapter, which focuses on the extensive diaries of Alice Slythe, a TFNS nurse who worked on the western front.[31] The diaries contain episode after episode in which Slythe describes her tourist activities while working as a nurse at a base hospital in Wimereux. Presented almost as a travel journal for the uninitiated (the diaries are addressed to Maud, her older sister), these descriptions of the sights and sounds of wartime France are punctuated by photographs, picture postcards, and other souvenirs. When Slythe moves up the line to a Casualty Clearing Station close to the front, her tourist activities become more adventurous, including trips to frontline trenches and episodes in which she and her colleagues narrowly avoid German shelling. However, the diaries are also punctuated by episodes in which the mood changes and the diaries begin to engage with what she calls "horrors," traumatic injury, suffering, and death.[32] In the later volumes, names of patients begin to appear and there is a sense that Slythe has become emotionally involved in her patients' sufferings and frustrated at the little she is able to do for certain hopeless cases. At this point Slythe expresses a horror of the war and reveals pacifist sentiments. Slythe provides us with a clear example of a nurse who had been trained to draw firm boundaries between her professional and personal lives, and who had already used her training to good effect in her previous nursing work, for example, when nursing casualties of railway accidents in London, an experience to which she refers in her diaries. Clearly proud of her competence as a trained nurse, she did not generally view her nursing work as suitable content for a personal diary, and she employed a degree of self-censorship. In addition, it was certainly the case that travel abroad during the war for many nurses did take on the nature of an adventure—especially taking into account the fact that northern France in 1914–1918 had become a meeting point for men and women of multiple nationalities and ethnicities. Despite this, the few passages that relate to her nursing practice reveal that her experiences in France were professionally challenging and, at times, emotionally draining.

The final part of the volume—"Nurse as Witness"—focuses on the unique perspective enjoyed by nurses as chroniclers of the war and its consequences. Nurses witnessed the war in a way that no other group could have witnessed it. Their perspective was that of closely involved participants in a destructive conflict, who were themselves neither destroyers nor destroyed, neither combatants nor wounded.[33] Santanu Das has written compellingly of the "impotence of sympathy" experienced by nurses, the extent to which their role compelled them to observe a suffering that they were powerless to prevent. His observation allows us to view nurses as trapped in the machinery of a war over which they had no power or influence.[34] Yet, in another sense, nurses were not simply passive observers. They had a well-defined role: they healed the wounds of war, they "patched up" the damaged bodies of their patients, and they offered support, both physical and emotional, to the men they nursed. Their perspectives thus differ, for example, from the testimony of the chaplains or civilian relatives who helplessly watched over the final hours of dying men. All of the chapters in this part reveal that nurses' perspectives on both the war itself and their role in it were often highly ambivalent. Yet, for the most part, they retained a conviction that they were making a positive contribution both to individual lives and to the war effort.

Carol Acton's chapter considers the ambivalence of the nurse–patient relationship in the writings of professional and VAD nurses. She argues that in the necessarily intimate relationship of nurses to wounded male bodies, nurse-writers were often caught between conflicting desires to articulate the damage to male bodies wrought by the war and to restore dignity to the wounded "heroes" by means of the romanticization of both their bodies and their wounds. Thus, their writings convey a sense that the nurse, in caring for the wounded, was in some sense participating in the heroism of war, yet the realities of horrific and ugly war-wounds created a deep tension between the mythic propaganda of war and the realities of bloody amputation stumps and disintegrating bodies. Acton frames this tension as a process of "negotiating masculinity," with the wound functioning simultaneously as a marker of masculinity and as evidence of the destructive nature of warfare. Another dilemma for the nurses whose autobiographical writings Acton draws on lay in the extent to which, as idealized "ministering angels," they attempted to steer a path between professional detachment and romantic—or even erotic—attachment to the men they nursed. For some writers, the failure to find an anticipated romance and heroism in their work resulted in contradiction and confusion; for others the process of writing about their experiences was in itself a confrontation with the realities of the First World War as a war of emasculation and annihilation.

The shifting and multiple perspectives of the volunteer nurse as witness to war are captured in all of their complexity by Hazel Hutchison in her analysis of American Mary Borden's writings. *The Forbidden Zone*, written mainly contemporaneously with Borden's wartime experiences, but reworked and published as a whole in 1929, has become one of the iconic modernist texts of the First World War, quoted both by scholars of wartime nursing for its attention to the detail of nursing practice and by literary critics for the consummate observation and writing skills displayed in it.[35] Hutchison argues that the power of the text ultimately derives from Borden's complex use of observation in many forms. Identifying herself primarily as a writer, and more particularly as a literary modernist, Borden is nevertheless also an American, a philanthropist, and the *Directrice* of a number of French field hospitals. The power of her writing emerges from observational skills that are, at different times, literary, clinical, managerial, detached, and involved. Occasional panoramic overviews of the war zone are juxtaposed with intimate descriptions of individual incidents, and wartime medical practice, which are captured with realism and precision. Her fragmentary style is imbued with an awareness and, ultimately, a critique of the impact of wartime violence on the bodies of individual men. Borden's work draws on the broad literary canon available to a well-educated American woman, and she effectively puts her knowledge and literary skills to work on a unique experience, creating a highly original and influential text.

The theme of observation in nurse memoirs is also addressed by Margaret Higonnet. Higonnet likens the autobiographical texts of some modernist nurse-writers—who were writing within a medical context in which technical innovations, such as the development of X-rays, had greatly enhanced the powers of observation—to the cubist art forms of the early twentieth century. Drawing on works of Americans Mary Borden and Ellen LaMotte, Russian Lidiia Zakharova, Italian Maria Luisa Perduca, and Romanian Hortensia Papadat Bengescu, Higonnet reveals the "multiplication of angles of perception" embodied in these writings.[36] As they deliberately "break up" our perspective, these texts aim at capturing a more profound version of the "truth" than a superficial, one-dimensional view can offer. Their works effectively demonstrate the many ways in which the hospital can become a place of theater and spectacle, with treatments and scenarios—including X-rays, surgical operations, and nurses' bedside vigils—that enable multiple viewpoints. In detailing the various ways in which what Michel Foucault termed the "medical gaze" can thus approach the body from a range of angles, Higonnet explores how some of the nurse-writers of the First World War used their positions as nurses to interrogate the moral dimensions and dilemmas of war, employing a range of planes and angles to get beneath and dissect its ethical complexities.

No study of nursing during the First World War can avoid being influenced by distortions in the historical record. The preservation of some sources and the loss or destruction of others—processes that are, themselves, dictated by the political and cultural choices of archivists, curators, and private individuals—mean that histories written in the twenty-first century are colored by layers of past engagement with the subject. The ways in which subsequent generations have chosen to preserve the memory of those who nursed during the war have influenced both "official" and "revisionist" histories of women and the First World War. Alison Fell's afterword addresses these issues, arguing that, from the 1920s onward, different generations in both Britain and France remembered nurses in distinct ways. Drawing on various forms of commemorative discourse, including war memorials, ceremonies, speeches, and the minutes of nursing and veteran organizations, Fell shows that in the 1920s, during the first period of memorialization, the commemoration of the war dead in both Britain and France tended to portray nursing as the female, nurturing counterbalance to the masculine, heroic combatant. By contrast, nursing organizations themselves, both volunteer and professional, preferred to portray their members as expert professionals playing a significant role in warfare, or as fallen heroines, who (albeit in smaller numbers than soldiers) placed themselves in danger and lost their lives in their pursuit of the Allied cause. In so doing they implicitly called for recognition and gratitude from their respective nations for their significant participation in the national "sacrifices" made during the conflict.

In the 1930s, in the context of the rise of a pacifist consciousness and the cultural emergence of an interpretation of the First World War as a deplorable and avoidable waste of life, the idea of the wartime nurse as reluctant witness to meaningless destruction took hold, a version of events that was associated in Britain with the publication of commercially successful books such as Vera Brittain's *Testament of Youth* and Irene Rathbone's

We That Were Young. Although other memoirs were published, this voice of the nurse as a female equivalent of the embittered veteran was the one that appeared to resonate most with the British public during the interwar years. However, new interpretations of First World War nursing emerged with the arrival of second-wave feminism in the 1970s. In Britain, popular cultural outputs, such as the Imperial War Museum's 1977 *Women at War* exhibition, with its accompanying book by Arthur Marwick, emphasized the ways in which the war provided a route for women to greater public engagement, freeing middle-class volunteer nurses from the backwater of domestic life.[37] In so doing, Marwick's book underplayed the role of trained nurses, and failed to take fully into account the grief and trauma experienced by some nurses who bore witness to the physical and psychological damage wrought by mechanized warfare. Subsequent contributions to the literature—particularly those of feminist writers—have both developed and countered some of the more simplistic elements of an argument that depicted war as "liberating" for volunteer nurses. Fell's afterword argues that these broad shifts in the public perception of the First World War nurse have influenced academic writing on the subject—including the chapters to be found in this volume, some of which point to the inherent ambiguities evident in the writings of volunteer nurses, and others of which emphasize a need to focus on the more neglected works of trained professional nurses.

Images of the nurse appeared everywhere during the First World War. They were frequent figures on postcards and posters, in newspapers and popular journals. To a large extent, an idealized version of the nurse—as devoted, caring, virtuous, and pure—was adopted in the Allied nations as the female equivalent of the mobilized man. Transnationally, the nurse was often used to embody abstract sentiments or qualities such as "Humanity";[38] nationally, the figure functioned more frequently as an icon of female patriotism and a call to arms for those still to be mobilized in the war effort. Although hospital work allowed some women to enter the militarized zone, normally out-of-bounds for women, nursing as an occupation was firmly situated within traditional understandings of women's roles as wives and mothers, and for this reason the nurse-as-icon had broad appeal. The Red Cross nurse in particular was a role model for many middle- and upper-class women seeking a respectable patriotic role in wartime Europe.[39] Yet this volume underlines the fact that nurses—in terms of the thousands of individual women who actually performed the role during the conflict—were the subjects as well as the objects of the gaze. And while popular images of the nurse tend to rely on well-worn and comforting clichés of femininity, the testimony of flesh-and-blood women offers a much more varied and often conflicted account of the roles, experiences, and perspectives of First World War nurses. As Margaret Higonnet reminds us, we frequently find a "multiplication of perceptions in the pursuit of new understanding in nurses' writings about the Great War."[40] Nurses' texts crystallize the liminal position in which women who were active during the First World War found themselves. Nurses, perhaps more than other female war workers, were obliged to perform what Dorothy Goldman calls the "different and complex double function" of women war writers, being simultaneously "actors in their own war and spectators of the soldiers' war."[41] Their texts often oscillate between these different perspectives, expressing their need to function as channels for lamenting the physical and psychological consequences of war alongside a desire to chronicle women's important contributions as vital components in the medical care and treatment of combatant patients. The hesitations that this brought about get to the heart of the ethical "double bind" of women asked to heal men in order that they be sent back to the front. Consequently, the chapters in this volume consistently suggest that a serious consideration of a broad corpus of the written texts produced by nurses from different Allied nations leads us, necessarily, to revise our understanding of the First World War, offering important new (and, inevitably, gendered) perspectives on the experiences and legacies of war.

NOTES

1. P. Fussell, *The Great War and Modern Memory* (Oxford: Oxford University Press, 2000 [1975]).
2. Later cultural histories focused, in particular, on the identities of combatants and on the memorialization of their sacrifice. See, for example, E. J. Leed, *No Man's Land: Combat and Identity in World War One* (New York: Cambridge University Press, 1979); M. Eckstein, *Rites of Spring: The Great War and the Birth of the Modern Age* (Boston: Houghton Mifflin Company, 1989); J. Winter, *Sites of Memory, Sites of Mourning: The Great War in European Cultural History* (Cambridge: Cambridge University Press, 1995).
3. C. M. Tylee, *The Great War and Women's Consciousness: Images of Militarism and Womanhood in Women's Writings, 1914–1964* (Houndmills: Macmillan, 1990); M. Higonnet et al., eds., *Behind the Lines: Gender and the Two World Wars* (New Haven, CT: Yale University Press, 1987); M. Higonnet, *Lines of Fire. Women Writers of World War I* (Harmondsworth: Penguin, 1999); M. Higonnet, *Nurses at the Front: Writing the Wounds of the Great War* (Boston: Northeastern University Press, 2001); M. Higonnet, "Authenticity and Art in Trauma Narratives of World War I," *Modernism/Modernity* 9, no. 1 (2002): 91–107; S. Ouditt, *Fighting Forces, Writing Women: Identity and Ideology in the First World War* (London: Routledge, 1994); A. K. Smith, *The Second Battlefield: Women, Modernism and the First World War* (Manchester: Manchester University Press, 2000).
4. On the formation of the British military nursing services, see A. Summers, *Angels and Citizens: British Women as Military Nurses, 1854–1914*, rev. ed. (Newbury, Berks: Threshold Press, 2000).
5. V. L. Holder, "From Hand-Maiden to Right Hand," *AORN Journal* 80, no. 4 (2004): 657.
6. T. Bowser, *The Story of British VAD Work in the Great War* (London: Imperial War Museum, 2003, facsimile of the 1917 ed.); Y. McEwen, *"It's a Long Way to Tipperary": British and Irish Nurses in the Great War* (Dunfermline: Cualann Press, 2006), 39, 99; L. Macdonald, *The Roses of No Man's Land*

(London: Michael Joseph, 1980), 29; Ouditt, *Fighting Forces*, 15. It should be noted that because of the inadequate surviving records of the different organizations to which nurses belonged, exact statistics remain difficult to establish.

7. See Chapters 3, 8, and 9.
8. K. Jensen, *Mobilizing Minerva: American Women in the First World War* (Urbana: University of Illinois Press, 2008), 120. On American nursing in the First World War, see also M. Sarnecky, *A History of the US Army Nurse Corps* (Philadelphia: University of Pennsylvania Press, 1999); J. Stimson, "The Army Nurse Corps," in F. Weed and L. McAfee, *The Medical Department of the United States Army in the World War* (Washington, DC: Government Printing Office, 1927), vol. 2: 125–8; S. Zeiger, *In Uncle Sam's Service: Women Workers with the American Expeditionary Forces, 1917–1919* (Ithaca, NY: Cornell University Press, 1999).
9. Y. Knibiehler, *Cornettes et blouses blanches: Les Infirmières dans la société française 1880–1980* (Paris: Hachette, 1984), 96.
10. The three organizations that made up the French Red Cross were: *La Société de Secours aux Blessés Militaires* (founded 1864), *L'Association des Dames Françaises* (founded 1877), and *L'Union des Femmes Françaises* (founded 1881).
11. F. Thébaud, *La Femme au temps de la guerre de 14* (Paris: Stock, 1986), 86; J-Y. Le Naour, *Misères et tourments de la chair durant la Grande Guerre* (Paris: Aubier, 2002), 75.
12. A. Lindenmeyr, *Poverty Is Not a Vice: Charity, Society and the State in Imperial Russia* (Princeton, NJ: Princeton University Press, 1996), 125–26.
13. V. P. Romaniuk, V. A. Lapotnikov, and Ia. A. Nakatis, *Istoriia sestrinskogo dela v Rossii* (Saint Petersburg: SPbGMA, 1998), 78. Quoted in http://russiasgreatwar.org/media/homefront/sisters_of_mercy.shtml.
14. A. Gibelli, *La Grande Guerra degli Italiani, 1915–1918* (Milan: Coen & C, 1998), 248. See also A. Scardino Belzer, "The Other Army: Italian Women on the Home Front during the First World War," *Minerva Journal of Women and War* 3, no. 1 (2009): 6–23.
15. See M. Bucur, "Women's Stories as Sites of Memory: Gender and Remembering Romania's World Wars," in *Gender and War in Twentieth-Century Eastern Europe*, ed. N. M. Wingfield and M. Bucur (Bloomington: Indiana University Press, 2006), 171–92. Bucur refers to Romanian Red Cross nurses who published their war memoirs in the 1920s, one of whom dedicated her memoirs to Queen Marie.
16. I. Petrović, "Foreign Medical Help in Serbian Liberation Wars from 1912 until 1918," *Arch Oncol* 18, no. 4 (2010): 143–48.
17. See Chapter 2.
18. For extracts from a British volunteer who worked at the Hôtel de l'Océan with Dr. Depage, see "Mrs. Elsie Fenwick," in *Women in the War Zone*, ed. A. Powell (Stroud: History Press, 2009), 130–40.
19. See, for example, *The British Journal of Nursing* (23 January 1915); *L'Illustration* (23 January 1915): 79; *The Times* (23 January 1915). See also G. Daniels, "Humanitarianism or Politics? Japanese Red Cross Nurses in Britain, 1915–1916," in *Japanese Women Emerging from Subservience*, ed. H. Tomida and G. Daniels (Folkestone: Global Oriental, 2005), 222–31.
20. L. Leneman, "Medical Women at War 1914–1918," *Medical History* 38 (1994): 160–77: 168.
21. See Chapter 6. These issues are discussed in C. Hallett, *Containing Trauma: Nursing Work in the First World War* (Manchester: Manchester University Press, 2009).
22. See Chapter 5.

23. Knibiehler, *Cornettes et blouses blanches*, 96–105; K. Schultheiss, *Bodies and Souls: Politics and the Professionalization of Nursing in France, 1880–1922* (Cambridge, MA: Harvard University Press, 2001).
24. Much recent scholarship on professional military nursing in World War I has emerged from Australia. See, for example, J. Bassett, *Guns and Brooches: Australian Army Nursing from the Boer War to the Gulf War* (Melbourne: Oxford University Press, 1992); R. Rae, *Veiled Lives. Threading Australian Nursing History into the Fabric of the First World War* (Burwood, NSW: College of Nursing, 2009); K. Harris, *More than Bombs and Bandages. Australian Army Nurses at Work in World War I* (Newport, NSW: Big Sky Publishing, 2010).
25. C. E. Hallett, "Portrayals of Suffering: Perceptions of Trauma in the Writings of First World War Nurses and Volunteers," *Canadian Bulletin of Medical History* 27, no. 1 (2011): 65–84.
26. Hallett, *Containing Trauma.*
27. C. E. Hallett, "The Personal Writings of First World War Nurses: A Study of the Interplay of Authorial Intention and Scholarly Interpretation," *Nursing Inquiry* 14, no. 4 (2007): 320–29.
28. I. Rathbone, *We That Were Young* (London: Virago Press, 1988 [1932]); V. Brittain, *Testament of Youth* (Glasgow: Collins and Sons, 1980 [1933]).
29. Rathbone, *We That Were Young.*
30. E. Bagnold, *A Diary without Dates* (London: Virago, 1978 [1918]).
31. A. Slythe, Diaries, Liddle Collection, University of Leeds, WO 107.
32. Ibid., 16 June 1916.
33. Though it should be noted that at least one thousand Allied nurses were killed as a direct result of their participation in the war or died from an illness contracted in service. Again, exact figures are difficult to establish. Many nurses' "war deaths" were due to influenza contracted in service toward the end of the war. British nurses who were injured were entitled to a military pension, and three hundred of their files (2 percent of the total) are available in the National Archives. They reveal that the contraction of diseases such as malaria or neurasthenia attributed to their war experiences continued to affect their lives for many years afterward. TNA, PIN 26/19985–PIN 26/22744.
34. S. Das, *Touch and Intimacy in First World War Literature* (Cambridge: Cambridge University Press, 2005).
35. M. Borden, *The Forbidden Zone*, ed. H. Hutchison (London: Hesperus Press, 2008).
36. For further insight into the works of these writers, see also Higonnet, *Lines of Fire.*
37. A. Marwick, *Women at War 1914–1918* (London: Fontana, 1977).
38. Edith Cavell is the most well-known example of this. See the afterword in this volume.
39. See A. S. Fell, "Nursing the Other: The Representation of Colonial Troops in French and British Nursing Memoirs," in *Race, Empire and First World War Writing*, ed. S. Das (Cambridge: Cambridge University Press, 2011), 158–74; M. Darrow, "French Volunteer Nursing and the Myth of War Experience in World War I," *American Historical Review* 101, no. 1 (1996): 80–106; Ouditt, *Fighting Forces*; Hallett, *Containing Trauma.*
40. See Chapter 9.
41. D. Goldman, *Women Writers and the Great War* (New York: Twayne, 1995), 102, quoted in A. S. Fell, "Myth, Countermyth and the Politics of Memory: Vera Brittain and Madeleine Clemenceau Jacquemaire's Interwar Nurse Memoirs," *Synergies* 4 (2011): 11–22.

Part I

National Identities

1 Making Sister Julie

The Origin of First World War French Nursing Heroines in Franco-Prussian War Stories

Margaret H. Darrow

In the fall of 1914, Sister Julie of Gerbéviller became a media heroine. According to the many press accounts and interviews, this sixty-one-year-old nun had confronted the invading German army and defeated it. The French press had begun to report her activities in early September; the story spread quickly, her exploits multiplying in each new iteration. Originally commended for her courage in nursing under bombardment, newspapers soon credited her with saving Gerbéviller from destruction and wounded French soldiers from massacre.[1] While some images transformed her into a slender young woman, many journalists delighted in describing her short, stout, pugnacious person: "her eyes sparkling, her whole face expressing kindness," "comely and fresh as an apple," "a tough, little, resourceful . . . countrywoman, full of goodness and practicality." "Lacking very scientific methods, [she] poured out the balm of her spirit, what her good sense told her was best to do." Everyone's granny and, according to Maurice Barrès, "all this enhanced by spirituality." "A soldier, in fact," a soldier "for God and for France."[2]

The France that Sister Julie embodied was not invaded and occupied but triumphant. Although accounts praised her nursing and her care for the poor and the refugees, the core of her story was the confrontation and defeat of the German invaders. Later versions of her tale multiplied the confrontations; British journalist White Williams, who interviewed her in 1915, related five separate incidents in which Sister Julie routed the Germans.[3] The confrontation most frequently recounted, and also illustrated (see Figure 1.1), occurred over the bodies of wounded French soldiers for whom she was caring. In early accounts, the German commander merely wanted to make them prisoners; in later ones, murder was his intent. In a 1917 interview, Sister Julie asserted that the officer had had a dagger hidden in his breast and his finger on the trigger of his pistol, meaning "to harm our poor little wounded." Pantomiming both parts in the confrontation, "she raises the poignard of the German Colonel; you see it held over her head ready to strike." Then she mimed throwing herself across the bed of a wounded soldier, saving his life and those of all the wounded. The vignette concluded with the German officer's capitulation—"Madame, you are brave; no one will harm you."[4]

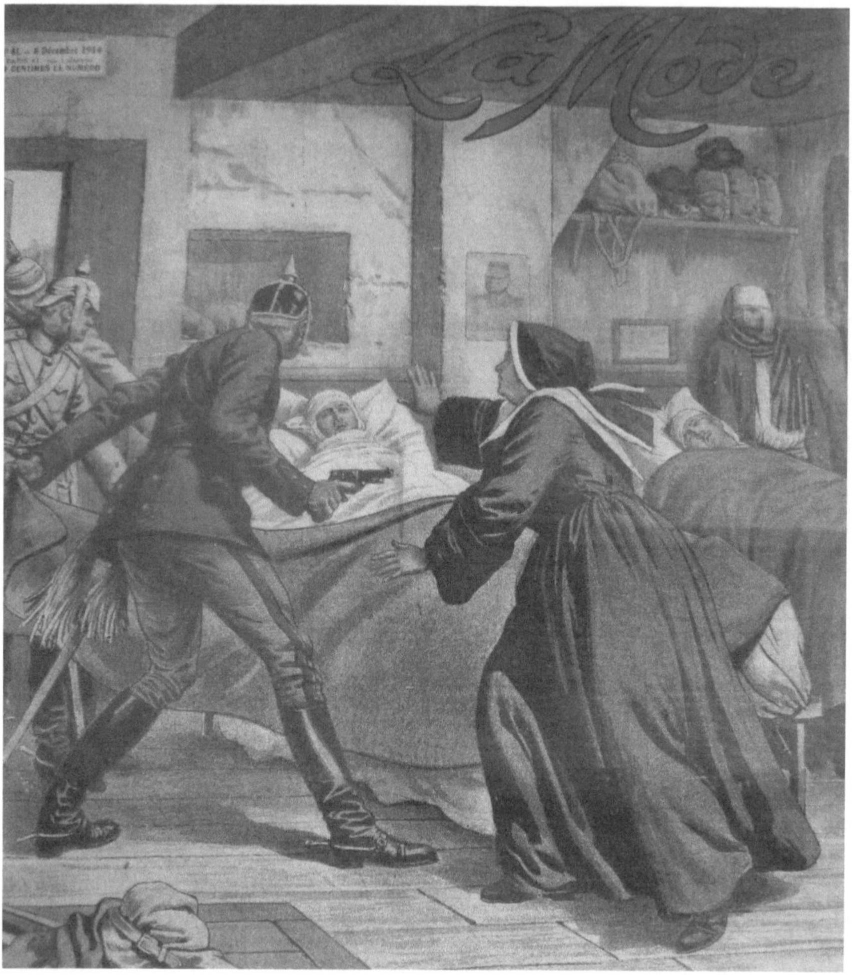

Figure 1.1 The cover of *La Mode* (6 December 1914). Sister Julie confronting the German menace, 24 August 1914. Courtesy of the Bibliothèque nationale de France.

In the first months of the war, Sister Julie was the best-known French nurse. But neither her actions nor her image derived from the Red Cross, the main source of French nurses during the war. In fact, Sister Julie, her person, and her actions, were nearly antithetical to the image of women's wartime nursing that the French Red Cross worked to convey: secular, professionally trained, under the authority of a male doctor, in an auxiliary hospital far from combat. Instead, Sister Julie's story rested on earlier models of French women's contributions to war. Although these models had antecedents in the Napoleonic Wars and even earlier, reports of French women's nursing in the Franco-Prussian War had recently updated and popularized them. Nursing stories from the Franco-Prussian War not only shaped the press reports of Sister Julie; they also influenced French women's response to the outbreak of war in 1914.

The role of the French Red Cross in the Franco-Prussian War, and the stories it inspired, was complicated, even conflicted. This was the first war in which the French Red Cross, founded in 1866, had participated.[5] On the one hand, it gained the young organization publicity and respect; on the other, the war revealed the organization's inadequacy. The latter view came to dominate in the two decades before 1914 as rival branches of the French Red Cross competed for members, money, and official recognition. The first French organization of the Red Cross, the Society to Aid the Military Wounded (Société de secours aux blessés militaires or SSBM),[6] was small, elitist, and all male. In the few years prior to the outbreak of the Franco-Prussian War its leadership hosted an international conference and organized an exhibit at the Exposition Universelle of 1867 but did little to expand the organization beyond the imperial court circle or prepare for practical wartime intervention. The outbreak of war in July 1870 found the SSMB with only three functioning branches and little in the way of medical staff, materials, or funds. Nonetheless, it quickly organized and dispatched sixteen ambulances from Paris to the front. Once Paris was besieged, the SSMB continued operations from the provinces, setting up and supplying emergency aid posts and hospitals as the German armies swept through northern and central France.[7]

During and immediately after the war, the SSMB received much praise for its efforts, but it quickly relapsed into inactivity. Two new Red Cross organizations—the Association des Dames françaises (ADF), founded in 1879 for women, and the Union des Femmes de France (UFF), founded in 1881 by women—revitalized the French Red Cross and gave it a new direction.[8] Unlike the SSBM, these societies recruited and trained women for wartime nursing. They also vigorously lobbied the government and the military to include Red Cross volunteers in war planning.[9] In pursuing these goals, the ADF and the UFF reconfigured the meaning of volunteer nursing in the Franco-Prussian War. According to their spokespeople and literature, French women's response to the war in 1870 had been seriously inadequate—good-hearted but wrongheaded—and, in their lack of preparation, nearly as responsible for the French defeat as was the French army. Dr. Auguste Duchaussoy, founder of the ADF, wrote in a manual for nurses' training in 1881 that the "bitter memory of our lack of foresight" in 1870 showed "that the best promptings of the heart cannot replace technical knowledge." Dr. Pierre Bouloumié, speaking at a UFF conference, maintained, "We must have the courage to say that not everyone did her duty, all her duty, in 1870, and that is precisely because no one was prepared."[10] The SSMB in the Franco-Prussian War was blameworthy rather than praiseworthy, its story a cautionary tale to inspire the government, the army, and French women to do better, much better, in the future.[11] And to do better, everyone must support the French women's Red Cross organizations.

The story of volunteer nursing efforts during the Franco-Prussian War, as crafted by the ADF and the UFF, emphasized women's lack of preparation for the war, particularly in contrast to the German Red Cross.[12] Their promoters applauded the outpouring of French women's charity in 1870 but at the same time denigrated its efficacy. Their favorite word to describe these volunteers was "improvised":

> At the moment of terrible awakening, everything had to be created, improvised. While the men sought to remedy the disastrous consequences of their culpable negligence, women throughout the whole land met in committees as soon as the war began, to organize everything that was needed, improvising tents, beds, bandages, medicine . . . It is not easy to create an administration, to improvise facilities and all this in the midst of a terrible crisis like the one then taking place in France.[13]

Such a situation should not occur again. As journalist Maxime Du Camp wrote in his three-part article on the Red Cross in *La Revue des deux mondes*: "Never again should we be caught unprepared by events, as we were in July 1870, having to organize in the midst of battle, in the face of the enemy."[14]

In their 1912 book, *La Femme sur le champ de bataille*, Dr. Arnaud and Dr. Bonnette divided women's wartime nursing into two types, the "improvised nurses" of the past and the professionally trained volunteers that they advocated for the future: "By *improvised nurses* we mean women whom wartime chance has abruptly placed before the wounded or ill, and who display all the treasures of charity and devotion until then hidden in their nature."[15] Ste Hélène, Paulette Bonaparte, Sisters of Charity, "society ladies and bourgeoisies," *cantinières*,[16] and actresses, Dr. Arnaud and Dr. Bonnette described them all in the same terms: their hearts were in the right place but they were untrained and unorganized. Modern warfare demanded more than Christian charity, *noblesse oblige*, and maternal instinct. "In modern wars we no longer find the nun or the *cantinière*, as in the past, stooping to ease or bandage the wounded. These different feminine types have both disappeared." They were replaced, the authors asserted, by the "vocational nurse," scientifically trained and professionally experienced: "we mean the French Red Cross."[17] At this point, the book reveals its true character: a recruiting tract for the Red Cross. Dr. Arnaud and Dr. Bonnette exhort French women to prepare now for their future wartime duty.

Other Red Cross promoters went further in their criticism of volunteer nursing in the Franco-Prussian War and in their recipes for improvement. Dr. Eifer, an ADF supporter, ridiculed the much-publicized hospital that the Comédie Française had set up in 1870 as amateurish and even frivolous: "You don't improvise a nurse any more than you improvise an actress; each career requires a long apprenticeship," he claimed.[18] The appropriate model, according to Maxime Du Camp, was the army; just as soldiers trained in anticipation of war, so should volunteer nurses. "In a country where the armies are permanent and always in a state of readiness, the societies responsible for medical services must be similarly permanent."[19]

Among the variety of improvised nurses that Red Cross promoters denigrated were most of the volunteer nurses of the Franco-Prussian War. While the historic examples that Arnaud and Bonnette cited, like Ste Hélène, were scarcely rivals to the contemporary Red Cross, the Franco-Prussian War nurses were, and although they would be overshadowed and forgotten in the Red Cross's triumph in the First World War, their stories were quite familiar to French women in the years prior to 1914. In fact only the *cantinière* had truly disappeared, discontinued by the French army in 1905.[20] Stories of the others—Sisters of Charity, society ladies, *bourgeoisies*, and actresses—continued to inspire French women in 1914. These stories also served as models for press reports about nurses in the early months of the First World War.

Arnaud and Bonnette's 1912 list of improvised, outmoded nurses echoed the categories that publicists had developed not to denigrate but to celebrate French women's patriotism during the Franco-Prussian War. Paul and Henry de Trailles's compendium, *Les Femmes de France pendant la guerre et les deux sièges de Paris*, published in 1872, includes chapters titled "The Sister of Charity," "The Actress," "The Cantinière," and "The Society Lady," as well as "The Ambulance Nurse."[21] This variety really boiled down to two sorts of activity. Ladies and actresses created, administered, and nursed in auxiliary hospitals; *cantinières* and ambulance nurses tended the wounded on or near the battlefield. Sisters of Charity could figure in either role.

As early as 19 July 1870, the day war was declared, *La Petite Presse* reported, under the title "Women under the Colors!", that "a certain number of ladies request authorization to follow the troops in the eventuality of war, to lavish their care in the ambulances." A week later the paper reported, "The number of ladies who ask to go to the ambulances is greater and greater . . . in fact, we have heard there are now nearly a thousand such requests."[22] All were directed to the Red Cross, but the SSBM limited women's contribution to collecting money and bed linen and making bandages. The society's president, the comte de Flavigny, dismissed such requests, implying that these women only wanted to follow their husbands or lovers.[23]

In mid-August reports appeared of a new direction to women's efforts. No longer asking permission to go with the troops, women were now setting up their own infirmaries and auxiliary hospitals and soliciting wounded be sent to them. Newspapers printed Baroness Rothschild's letter to the Minister of War, announcing that she was turning her château into an auxiliary hospital, and other well-to-do women quickly followed suit.[24] Organizations in Paris such as the Senate, the railroad companies, and even fashion houses turned their premises into auxiliary hospitals. Couturier Charles Frederick Worth, dressmaker to Empress Eugénie as well as most of fashionable Paris, opened a twenty-five-bed infirmary in his workrooms. Newspapers reported that the wives and daughters of these organizations' leaders were volunteering as nurses and nurses' aides.[25] In November, *Le Gaulois* recorded that in Paris's eighth arrondissement alone there were twenty-eight infirmaries, including three run by the military, several run by religious orders, and others by individuals like the duchesse de Chevreuse, Mme Pape-Charpentier, and Mme Dumoulins-Froment.[26] All of these, however, were upstaged when, during the siege of Paris, the Comédie Française and the Odéon Theater created infirmaries in their lobbies. Journalists made much of actresses like Madeleine Brohan, Marie Favart, Edile Riquier, and Sarah Bernhardt who had exchanged their theatrical roles, so the press claimed, for the "role of devotion" at the bedside of wounded soldiers.[27]

During and immediately after the war some commentators criticized these efforts much as the Red Cross did later. According to one doctor, these improvised hospitals were "without a doubt organized with much zeal but too often in naive ignorance of the conditions required for treating the wounded. . . . To attain this result, long study and a perfect knowledge of anatomy are necessary," not simply feminine solicitude. A newspaper columnist claimed that the society ladies who chatted about "my wounded" at their parties assigned the real work to their servants while they garnered the praise.[28] The most important of these critics was Dr. Léon Le Fort, a military surgeon who wrote a scathing condemnation of the SSBM's war work that included several sideswipes at volunteer nurses. It was their independence and their ambition as much as their ignorance of medicine that raised his hackles: "To wear a [Red Cross] arm band was, for some ladies, what a ribbon [of the Legion of Honor] is for many men. To have her own hospital became the fashionable ideal and some ladies played doctor with our poor soldiers like little girls play Mommy with their dolls."[29]

But both during and after the war, most of the writing about French women's efforts to set up and staff hospitals was extremely laudatory. Patronesses like the comtesse de Gouvion Saint-Cyr came in for extravagant praise: "She attended all the surgical operations; when an operation was particularly painful, she herself held the patient's hands in her own, while speaking words of encouragement that women know so well how to say. . . . Who, then, would not bow with respect before such magnanimity?"[30] Commentators marveled at the self-abnegation of actresses like Sarah Bernhardt: "What could be more touching than this famous woman who moves crowds with her words, whose least gesture unleashes tempests . . . and who, in the sacred name of the fatherland, throws away all her bouquets and, with cup in hand, quenches a poor soldier's thirst and spreads balm on his wound?"[31] Even ladies who visited the hospitals merely to hand out chocolates and smiles received commendation:

> They stop at each bed, seeking to console those with the most serious wounds and to raise their morale, their kind words go to the heart, their smiles comfort, and long after this brilliant apparition has disappeared, the poor wounded soldier still hears resonating in his ear that soft and charming voice that allowed him to forget his pain for a time.[32]

Besides the outpouring of praise from the press, there was also official recognition of women's wartime nursing as patriotic service. Mme Frary-Gross, who headed the hospital at the Hôtel de Ville, and Coralie Cahen, to whose story we will return, both received the Legion of Honor in recognition of their wartime work as did several Sisters of Charity.[33]

The decades following the war saw the publication of a number of compendia that recorded and celebrated French women's contributions to the national defense in 1870–1871. Although the first of these, Paul and Henry de Trailles's *Les Femmes de France pendant la guerre et les deux sièges de Paris*, appeared immediately after the war, the genre saw a resurgence in the late 1880s and 1890s beginning with the publication in 1887 of Jeanne France's *Les Femmes françaises pendant la guerre*, a compilation of supposedly true and admittedly fictional patriotic stories. Joseph Turquan's *1870–1871: Les Femmes de France pendant l'invasion*, published in 1893, and Ludovic Jablonski's *Les Femmes françaises à la guerre* in 1894 claimed to report only true stories. Among the heroines that they praised were Antoinette Lix, a *franc-tireur*, and Juliette Dodu, a telegraph operator, but most were nurses. Alexandre Piédagnel's *Les Ambulances de Paris pendant le siège* (1871) and Maxime Du Camp's *Paris Bienfaisant* (1888) catalogued and honored the many volunteer infirmaries that Parisiennes had run during the siege; Piédagnel described thirty-three of them in detail and included an index of the main personnel involved. General Ambert's popular history of the war, *Gaulois et Germains: Récits militaires*, included long excerpts from Piédagnel, further publicizing women's volunteer nursing as did Sarah Bernhardt's self-congratulatory account in her 1907 memoirs.[34] These publications as well as magazine and newspaper articles left French women in no doubt that women's creation of, and work in, temporary hospitals during the war had been necessary and valued.[35]

These compendia also celebrated volunteer nursing on and near the battlefields of the Franco-Prussian War. While the women who founded and staffed auxiliary hospitals demonstrated patriotic charity and self-sacrifice, stories of battlefield nursing were about courage and, in the most renowned cases, triumph. Although some accounts of the courage of battlefield nurses emerged during the war,[36] most appeared in its aftermath, first in accounts of the war like that of General Ambert and then repeated and elaborated in the press and in collections of war stories.[37] Some, like the story of Sister Remoud, who refused to leave the side of a dying officer even as bullets ricocheted around her, simply honored nurses' courage under fire.[38] Others celebrated the "martyrdom" of Sisters of Charity who died on the battlefield as they tried to reach the wounded.[39] Going a step further, some accounts depicted nurses as the victims of German malevolence, as "Prussian" officers insulted, threatened, harassed, and even executed them for their devotion to French wounded.[40] The most frequently retold stories, however, were those in which the nurse met and defeated German barbarity, demonstrating the moral superiority of French civilization. Such were the stories of Sister Saint-Henri of Janville, Sister Jeanne de Chantal of Châteaudun, and Mme Coralie Cahen.

The story of Sister Saint-Henri was brief but set the stage for the more baroque tales of Sister Jeanne de Chantal and Mme Cahen. Superior of a small hospice in Janville, she insisted that a convoy of wounded French prisoners stop and be unloaded for treatment despite the Prussian officer's command that it move on. General Ambert quoted Captain André de Maricourt, a witness to the scene, to describe the dramatic confrontation between Prussian inhumanity and French charity:

> "No sir!" she cried energetically, "these wounded don't belong to you, they are mine; I don't want them dragged farther!" The Prussian tried to protest. "Enough!" this elderly nun declared imperiously. "Let's go, wagoneer, unharness your horses, and you, Sir, who want to make these wounded suffer unnecessarily, you are a scoundrel!" She was magnificent in her indignation and I believed I could see the spirit of France soaring over our heads.[41]

Later accounts concluded that as a result "the life of more than one of these unhappy soldiers was saved."[42] Paul Grolleron, a painter of touching and heroic military scenes, immortalized this episode on a canvas displayed at the 1888 Salon (see figure 1.2).[43]

Named in religion for an early seventeenth-century saint, Jeanne de Chantal was the superior of a convent in Châteaudun.[44] During the siege of that town, she and the other nuns nursed the wounded, but after the town was taken, according to some accounts, she intervened repeatedly with the German command. She defended the local priest accused of having a weapon in his house, she secured the release of hostages taken after an alleged sniper attack, and she prevented the bombardment of the town as reprisal for guerilla activity. Her most widely credited act was to throw herself in front of national guardsmen, accused of being *franc-tireurs*, to prevent their execution. According to Jeanne France's dramatic version of the story:

> [Jeanne de Chantal] walked with a firm step toward the Prussian officer. She was dressed in black, a white bonnet and black veil covered her head; she was a nun, about fifty years old, the head of the hospital. "Please wait a moment, sir," she said, "I have something to propose to you." Then she said quite simply, "Would you see any inconvenience,

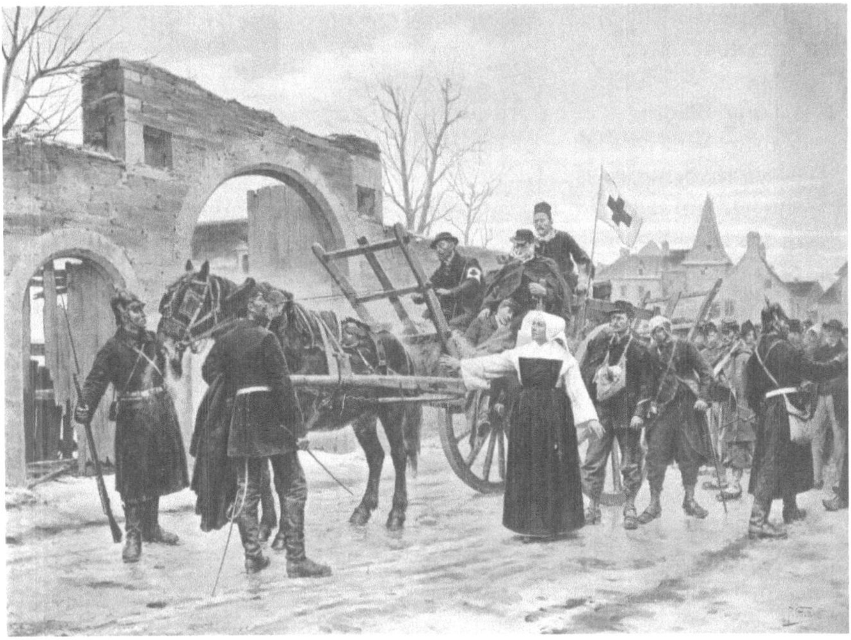

Figure 1.2 Sister Saint-Henri confronting the Prussian menace, as depicted by Paul Grolleron, 1888. Courtesy of the Bibliothèque nationale de France.

> sir, if I should be shot in place of these two men?" "But Madame . . ." stuttered the officer, completely taken aback. "You have said that it is necessary to make an example for the surrounding villages . . . Without boasting, I believe that the impression will be much stronger if you shoot a woman, a nun . . . Men shot in war, that happens every day." And she calmly walked to the execution post. "Stop!" cried the officer, deeply moved. "Good heavens, she is going to do it." "Be happy," he exclaimed as he approached her, "Because of you, I'll pardon those two . . . It would be a crime to kill so heroic a creature as you."[45]

In other accounts, Jeanne de Chantal is young, twenty-five years old rather than fifty, and the number of guerilla fighters she saved varies from story to story. However, the dramatic confrontation and the Prussian officer's capitulation to her bravery are the key episodes in all.[46]

Beside these stories of nun-heroines stood that of Mme Coralie Cahen, a Jewish widow. She began her wartime nursing in Metz, where, under the auspices of the French Red Cross, she organized the collection of wounded from the battlefields. With the help of other Metz ladies, she set up and ran an infirmary to care for them. Drawing on her close ties to the Rothchild's, she obtained credit to fund the Red Cross in Metz when it was cut off from the rest of France by the German siege. Even Dr. Le Fort, a bitter critic of the SSBM, grudgingly exempted her from his condemnation of volunteer nurses:

> I would be guilty of ingratitude if I did not make an exception for Mme Cahen. Widow of one of our most estimable colleagues, she came to Metz to bring to the wounded in our hospitals the long experience she had gained in supervising and directing several medical establishments founded by the Jewish community of Paris . . . she was the savior of the Fabert Hospital, by her unremitting and active supervision of the subordinate personnel, by herself directing the distribution of food and medicine, by presiding over the laundry, by lavishing upon our poor wounded and sick soldiers the consolation and soft words that are known to women's hearts alone.[47]

When Metz fell, she went to Vendôme, again at the behest of the SSBM, to set up another temporary hospital. After the war, she visited French POWs in Germany, bringing back copies of German records that established the fate of many soldiers missing in action. For her humanitarian work, in 1888 the French government awarded her the Legion of Honor.[48]

The central exploit of her story was her confrontation with a German general.[49] Having captured Vendôme, he had a Prussian flag raised over her infirmary. When she protested that her infirmary was, and would remain, French, he dismissed her with the boast: "We are masters here!" She replied: "In the town, maybe, but here, no! We are covered by the Red Cross and the French flag, and you have no right to touch one or the other" and threatened to close the facility, which was treating German as well as French wounded, if the Prussian flag did not come down immediately. He agreed, but as a favor to her in return for her care of German wounded, but she was having none of his favors; she insisted that he acknowledge her moral authority, which, according to the account, in the end, he did. "You are right, Madame, he added simply, perhaps that is just" and had the flag removed. The accounts claimed that when the Germans finally left Vendôme, they saluted her: "We will never forget that you forced us to bow both before your patriotism and your charity."[50]

In stories of Sister Saint-Henri, Sister Jeanne de Chantal, and Mme Cahen, it is easy to see the roots of Sister Julie's story in 1914: the French woman courageously intervening to save French soldiers, confronting German militarism and defeating it.[51] In these stories, not only did the German officers back down; they ratified the women's action with their admiration. We find this trope in other stories of Franco-Prussian War heroines, like that of telegraph operator Juliette Dodu. According to the story, she was condemned to death for tapping into the German telegraph wires. However the Prussian Prince Frederick Charles, impressed by her bravery and patriotism, pardoned her, declaring: "Gentlemen, I hope there are many German women like this French woman."[52] Historian Stéphane Tison has found that speeches at ceremonies commemorating Franco-Prussian War battles often cited German commentary as evidence of French bravery. Admiration from the victorious enemy, he concludes, was the ultimate legitimation.[53]

In the autumn of 1914, as in the interwar period, this tale reconfigured defeat as victory. In a 1889 poem at once celebrating Sister Saint-Henri's bravery and Grolleron's depiction of it, Marius Grillet described the captured French soldiers as "wounded, feet bloody, heads hanging, ashamed . . . weary and dishonored," reflecting the fate of France until the nun-heroine stepped in to reverse the situation. "A holy anger, a holy pity / Suddenly rises up in this frail woman's heart / To master this conqueror."[54] Similarly, Mme Cahen's story demonstrated France's superiority "even if," as Cahen admitted, on the battlefield "we could not be victorious."[55] General Ambert claimed this moral victory for all French women: "While the citizen gave in to force and bowed before the conqueror, the woman, with her head held high and a disdainful look, weighed up the German. The man exchanged a few more or less courteous words with her; the woman kept silent. She was, truly, the mute image of the fatherland."[56] In 1914, however, with the war still in progress, Sister Julie's story went further than demonstrating France's superiority to German barbarism; it held out the promise that her moral victory would soon be completed by a military one.

However, the Sister Julie story is not simply a repetition of these Franco-Prussian War stories; it is a reworking of them, imparting new meaning to some elements and passing over others in silence. One element that figured, although not prominently, in the accounts of Sister Saint-Henri and Mme Cahen that had little place in Sister Julie's story was their care for German as well as French wounded. After the war, the German monarchy recognized each nurse's work; Empress Augusta gave Cahen a Red Cross medal, while the emperor awarded Sister Saint-Henri eight thousand francs.[57] In her memoirs, Cahen explained she had made no distinction between French and German wounded "at first from strict humanitarianism and then, I must also say, for a sense of national dignity."[58] Such neutrality, of course, was central to the charter of the International Red Cross. However, as Rachel Chrastil has argued, after the mid-1880s, the French Red Cross hardly gave lip service to it; patriotism rather than humanitarianism dominated the rhetoric of all three organizations.[59] Sister Julie was not to be a heroine of neutrality; according to one article, "she recognized the right to prefer our wounded."[60]

Religion also functions differently in these tales. All four strongly marked the religious identity of the protagonists: three Catholic nuns and one Jewish widow. In the stories of Sister Saint-Henri and Sister Jeanne de Chantal, religion played a partisan role. By contrast, Mme Cahen's and Sister Julie's stories present their religion as a site of national reconciliation and unity.

The nun-heroine stories of the Franco-Prussian War were implicitly and sometimes explicitly partisan. While the secular press focused on their confrontations with the German army, Catholic accounts added details that identified them also as combatants for the Church against the republic.

They pointed out, for example, that despite "her services in the war with Germany," the republic's anticlerical campaign had driven Sister Jeanne de Chantal from her convent.[61] Sister Saint-Henri came in for praise for endowing a chapel, erecting a statue of Joan of Arc, and especially for her deathbed nursing of the resolute antirepublican Henri de Verthamon, standard-bearer of the Sacred Heart.[62] Abbé F. J. d'Ezerville's text, *Nos bonnes religieuses françaises . . . pendant la guerre de 1871*, claimed that all of the nuns who had nursed during the war were "admirable examples of patriotism and devotion to the national cause," living evidence of Catholicism's dominion and a rebuke to the republic's anticlericalism.[63] According to other Catholic writers, nuns had heroically sought out the wounded on the battlefield and nursed them when everyone else decamped. These accounts belittled the nursing of "ladies" as mere "advertising by the Jewish and anti-clerical press."[64] While Red Cross promoters tried to consign nuns to the unenlightened past of "improvised" war nursing, Catholic spokesmen claimed that *only* nuns had the qualities of patience, obedience, and self-abnegation as well as the moral authority necessary for ambulance work. The Red Cross, according to militant Catholic journalist Louis Veuillot, was an anticlerical republican plot to be resisted at all costs.[65]

By contrast, in the decades prior to the First World War, Coralie Cahen's story represented patriotic unity. All of the press coverage and commentary about Cahen's wartime activities underlined her identity as an "Israelite" and most drew a lesson from this. As Maxime Du Camp wrote in *La Revue des deux mondes* in 1888, her story must lay to rest any doubts "that the Israelites have only an incomplete commitment to the Fatherland."[66] In her own account, Cahen did more than claim patriotism for French Jews, she depicted an ethic and practice of devotion that united all French women in the national cause. She called attention to and praised the Catholic nuns who worked with her. She was moved and honored when they called her "mother" as they would their superior.[67] Such was her "sublime" devotion and her "ardent" patriotism that she was an example for all, according to Jacques Normand, reviewer for *La Revue bleue*; he wagered "that she would find favor even from the ferocious [anti-Semite] M. Drumont."[68]

It was from this legacy of reconciliation and unity rather than the partisan messages of the nun-heroines that chroniclers drew the meaning of Sister Julie's story. In these accounts, Sister Julie's religious status signified the reconciliation at last of the Church and the republic. Over the title "L'Union Sacrée," the cover of *J'ai vu* of 20 May 1916 displayed Sister Julie and anticlerical politician Emile Combes apparently side by side. Sister Julie, like the war's transcendent heroine, Joan of Arc, brought the two Frances finally together in an outpouring of patriotism.

By presenting visions of French moral superiority and national unity, the stories of Mme Cahen and Sister Julie boosted public morale. They carried an additional message for French women: that women's contribution was crucial to the national defense. This was, of course, the message of the Red

Cross campaign in the interwar years, but all of these stories celebrated examples of women's activities not sanctioned by the Red Cross. Sister Saint-Henri, Sister Jeanne de Chantal, and Mme Cahen demonstrated that French women, although untrained in medicine but endowed with feminine courage and maternal instinct, had played vital roles in the war zone in the recent past; Sister Julie's story carried this message into the present. Despite Red Cross admonitions that women had no business on the battlefield, in 1914 women flooded the Red Cross and the Ministry of War with requests to nurse in combat. Women as diverse as *bourgeoise* Julie Crémieux, actress Lola Noyr, and journalist Maria Lera believed that this was their patriotic duty. Noyr wrote in her memoirs, "I always wanted to go to the front; I considered that I was like a soldier and that to stay in the rear was to be rather like a shirker." They were frustrated and angry when they were rebuffed.[69]

Modeling themselves on the society women and actresses of 1870, well-to-do women with town houses and châteaux in 1914 hastened to offer them as auxiliary hospitals that they proposed to fund and run. In early August, the Marquise de Foucault wrote to Mme de Haussonville, president of the women's committee of the SSBM, to offer her château in Picardy as a hospital and reported that many of her acquaintances were doing the same.[70] Some, like the Duchesse d'Uzès, who turned her château at Rambouillet into a surgical unit,[71] had nursing certificates from the Red Cross; many, like the Marquise, did not. In his postwar memoirs, Dr. Lejars, head of the Villemin military hospital in Paris, snorted that most of these offers were the result of snobbery rather than patriotism and certainly not from any knowledge of what was necessary to treat wounded soldiers.[72] He was mostly correct in the second part of his criticism, but in his dismissal of patriotism as a motivation he ignored the precedent of the Franco-Prussian War. Officials at the beginning of the war, however, did remember. While they requested that unqualified women should stop volunteering to nurse, they also publicized infirmaries that well-to-do women were setting up.[73] Reports from Prefects around the country praised local *grandes dames* for their efforts to create auxiliary hospitals.[74]

A causal connection between the Franco-Prussian War nursing stories that proliferated in the 1890s and 1900s and French women's efforts to volunteer as nurses in 1914 can only be speculation. None of the French volunteer nurses who wrote accounts of their experiences explicitly refer to the Franco-Prussian War as an inspiration or mention any of that war's heroine nurses. The Red Cross received the credit for the deluge of women's volunteering in 1914, both at the time and since. The Red Cross campaign to define nursing as a female wartime duty equivalent to male military service was certainly largely responsible. However, French women's experience in the Franco-Prussian War and the publicity those efforts received in the intervening decades must also have played a role. Despite its campaign condemning "improvised" nurses, the Red Cross had not convinced all French women, or even all French authorities, that professionalism was more important than patriotism in a national crisis. In 1914 French women wanted to set up and run their own hospitals and to nurse on the battlefield. The stories of the Franco-Prussian War had shown them the way.

NOTES

1. Bibliothèque Marguerite Durand, 940.3 HER Guerre 1914–18 héroïnes; J.-M. Binot, *Héroïnes de la Grande Guerre* (Paris: Fayard, 2008), 29–40.
2. Dr. M. Delmas, "Comment Soeur Julie sauva son hôpital et ses blessés," *La Croix des Landes* (20 December 1914); W. Williams, "Soeur Julie de Gerbéviller," *La Guerre des nations: revue bimensuelle* 9 (1915); P. Romangy, "Soeur Julie," *La Mode illustrée: journal de famille* 56, no. 2 (10 January 1915): 16; Anonymous, "La Cornette protectrice des blessés: Sœur Julie de Gerbéviller," *Lectures pour tous* (15 January 1916); M. Barrès, "L'âme des ruines," *Echo de Paris* (4 November 1914); Anonymous, "Visite d'un journaliste parisien," *Le Petit Parisien* (29 September 1914); Anonymous, "Quelques exploits," *Echo de Paris* (27 December 1914).
3. Williams, "Soeur Julie." Also see "Soeur Julie," *La Mode* 41, no. 2 (6 December 1914): 594; R. B. Merriman, "A Day at the French Front," *Harvard Graduates Magazine* 24 (September 1915): 222–27.
4. A. Gleason, *Our Part in the Great War* (New York: Frederick A. Stokes Co., 1917), 294–317. Also see E. Wharton, *Fighting France from Dunkerque to Belfort* (New York: Charles Scribner's Sons, 1919), 102–4.
5. On the history of the French Red Cross, see V. Harouel, *Histoire de la Croix-Rouge* (Paris: Presses Universitaires de France, 1999); Knibiehler, *Cornettes et blouses blanches*; L. Ruault, *Cent ans de Croix-Rouge Française au service de l'humanité* (Paris: Hachette, 1964).
6. The full name was the Société de secours aux blessés militaires des armées de terre et de mer.
7. For an account of medical care during the war, especially in Paris, see B. Taithe, *Defeated Flesh: Welfare, Warfare and the Making of Modern France* (Manchester: Manchester University Press, 1999).
8. J. F. Hutchinson, *Champions of Charity: War and the Rise of the Red Cross* (Boulder, CO: Westview Press, 1996), 257.
9. On the French Red Cross organizations and campaigns prior to the First World War, see R. Chrastil, *Organizing for War: France 1870–1914* (Baton Rouge: Louisiana State University Press, 2010), 127–51; M. H. Darrow, *French Women and the First World War: War Stories of the Home Front* (Oxford: Berg, 2000), 28–30.
10. Dr. A. Duchaussoy, "Introduction," *L'Ecole des ambulancières et des garde-malades*, 4th ed. (Paris: Association des Dames françaises, 1906), iii; Dr. P. Bouloumié, *Union des Femmes de France, conférence à Lyon le 3 avril 1886* (Paris: Coopération typographique, 1886), 25. Bouloumié was a founder of the UDF and one of the very few men on its administrative board.
11. F. de Witt-Guizot, *La Femme et la guerre: Comment une femme peut-elle servir la France en temps de guerre?* (Autun: Imprimerie Pernot, 1913), 22; A. d'Alix, *La Croix-rouge française. Le rôle patriotique de femmes* (Paris: Perrin et cie., 1914), 37–38.
12. Military doctors and Red Cross promoters L. Arnaud and P. Bonnette, in *La Femme sur le champ de bataille* (Paris: Henri Charles-Lavauzelle, 1912), 91, cited these resources of the German Red Cross in 1870: official patronage,

two thousand local committees, seventy million francs in its war chest, and evacuation trains, "real rolling hospitals that moved 900 patients at a time to hospitals in home territory."

13. J. Turquan, *1870–1871: Les femmes de France pendant l'invasion* (Paris: Berger-Levrault et cie., 1893), 156–57. Gustave Moynier, a SSBN promoter, in *La Croix-Rouge: son passé et son avenir* (Paris: Sandoz and Thuillier, 1882), 78–79, concluded "an improvised medical service is not worth anything; so good sense tells us and the facts prove it. After the terrible experiences of 1870, we have seen that the [Red Cross] organizations in the former combatant countries and several neutral countries decided to make preparations that they rued having previously much neglected."
14. M. Du Camp, "La Croix-rouge de France," part 2, *Revue des deux mondes* 58, 90 (15 November 1888): 260–61. Du Camp concluded, "It was necessary to improvise everything" (273).
15. Arnaud and Bonnette, *La Femme*, 25; italics in text.
16. Cantinières were women licensed by the army to peddle food and drink to the soldiers. They were often the wives or daughters of noncommissioned officers. In the mid-nineteenth century, the cantinière was a celebrated figure. Dressed in a skirted uniform with a small keg of brandy slung from her shoulder, she accompanied the regiment on parade. During battles, she dispensed brandy, bandaged the wounded, and in a pinch fought alongside the soldiers. See T. Cardoza, *Intrepid Women: Cantinières and Vivandières of the French Army* (Bloomington: Indiana University Press, 2010).
17. Arnaud and Bonnette, *La Femme*, 84. Also see Dr. C. Legrand, *L'Assistance féminine en temps de guerre* (Paris: Librairie universelle, 1907), 263, 270.
18. Dr. Eifer, "Causerie Médicale: Nos ambulancières en temps de guerre," *La Femme de l'avenir* (1 October 1899).
19. Du Camp, "La Croix-rouge de France," part 1, *Revue des deux mondes* 58, 89 (15 October 1888): 751. In arguing for peacetime training for volunteer nurses, Dr. Duchaussoy made the same point: "you don't improvise good nurses any more than you do good soldiers" (*Ecole des ambulancières*, iii).
20. Cardoza, *Intrepid Women*, 210–14.
21. P. and H. de Trailles, *Les Femmes de France pendant la guerre et les deux sièges de Paris* (Paris: F. Polo Libraire-éditeur, 1872). Turquan also employs some of these categories.
22. *La Petite Presse* (19 July 1870); *La Petite Presse* (26 July 1870). On 30 July, the paper claimed that several hundred women every day requested to be placed as volunteers in ambulances.
23. *La Petite Presse* (25 July 1870).
24. *La Petite Presse* (16 August 1870).
25. *Le Gaulois* (28 August 1870); E. Charrier, *Croix-rouge. Union des Femmes de France: Paris 1914–15* (Paris: UFF, 1915).
26. *Le Gaulois* (21 November 1870).
27. *L'Illustration* (21 January 1871): 35; *La Petite Presse* (12 September 1870).
28. *Le Gaulois* (20 October 1870); *Journal des Débats* (27 February 1871). This accusation resurfaced in criticisms of volunteer nurses in the First World War. See Darrow, *French Women*, 146–48.
29. Dr. L. Le Fort, *La Chirurgie militaire et les sociétés de secours en France et à l'étranger* (Paris: Librairie Germer Baillière, 1872), 230. Le Fort was an aggrieved man. Initially asked by the SSBM to take charge of all its ambulances, the society's Central Committee later demoted him and stranded him in Metz without resources. This experience left him a bitter opponent of the Red Cross.
30. Turquan, *Les Femmes*, 164.

31. Ibid., 196, quoting General Ambert. For a similar panegyric to actresses as nurses, see Savigny, "L'Ambulance du Théâtre-Français," *L'Illustration* (21 January 1871): 35.
32. Turquan, *Les Femmes*, 190. Also see Trailles, *Les Femmes*, 61–62; A. Piédagnel, *Les Ambulances de Paris pendant le siège (1870–1871)* (Paris: Librairie générale, 1871).
33. A fascination with decorated women ensured that these honors were well publicized. See J. Alesson, *Les Femmes décorées de la légion d'honneur et les femmes militaires* (Paris: G. Melet libraire-editeur, 1886); A. de Valdor, "Les Femmes décorées," *La Femme et la famille* 57, no. 8 (August 1889): 233–35; H. Fontanges, *La Légion d'honneur et les femmes décorées* (Paris: Alliance coopérative du livre, 1905); "Cent neuf femmes légionnaires," *La Vie heureuse* (December 1905).
34. Général J. Ambert, *Gaulois et Germains: Récits militaires*, 4 vols. (Paris: Bloud et Barral, 1883–1885), 4:83–110; S. Bernhardt, *Ma double vie: mémoires de Sarah Bernhardt* (Paris: Charpentier et Fasquelle, 1907).
35. For example, de Valdor, "Les Femmes décorées," and the outpouring of laudatory obituaries for Coralie Cahen in March 1899.
36. *Le Gaulois* (17 August 1870).
37. See, for example, his praise for the women who nursed in Metz, "women from all classes: elegant ladies, modest *bourgeoises* and workers" (Ambert, *Gaulois et Germains*, 1:245).
38. Turquan, *Les Femmes*, 171–73; Arnaud and Bonnette, *La Femme*, 78.
39. Trailles, *Les Femmes*, 26–27; Abbé F. J. d'Ezerville, *Nos bonnes religieuses françaises: leurs états de service dans les classes, dans les orphelinats, dans les hôpitaux, pendant la guerre de 1871, près des vieillards* (Paris: Pené Haton, librairie-éditeur, 1877), 36–37.
40. Dr. E. Simonin, *Les Ambulances de Nancy en 1870 et 1871* (Nancy: Berger-Levrault, 1883), 80–81; d'Ezerville, *Nos bonnes religieuses*, 39–40; Dr. H. Dugast, *Souvenirs intimes de l'ambulance mobile de la Côte d'Or: Campagnes de la Loire et de l'Est, 1870–1871* (Dijon: J. Marchand, 1871), 31.
41. Ambert, *Gaulois et Germains*, 3, 135. De Maricourt published his own memoirs, *Casquettes blanches et croix rouge; Souvenirs de 1870: Coulmiers, Faverolles, Loigny, ambulances* (Paris: Firmin Didot, 1892), 181–82, that give a slightly different version of the story. Ambert's account, however, is the one that we see repeated in popular magazines, and, at Sister Saint-Henri's death, in her obituaries, for example, *Revue historique de l'Ouest* 6, no. 1 (1890): 231.
42. Turquan, *Les Femmes*, 174–77; Arnaud and Bonnette, *La Femme*, 78.
43. J. Richard, "Un convoi de blessés (Janville 1870)," *La Revue du siècle, littéraire, artistique & scientifique* 3, no. 3 (1889): 4–5, reproduced this painting and commented on it. Although Richard praised the realism and sentiment of the painting, he was skeptical of the story itself, suggesting it was fiction rather than history.
44. In the early seventeenth century François de Sales inspired Jeanne de Chantal to found a female religious order, the Order of the Visitation, whose main mission was to visit and comfort the sick, elderly, and poor. She was canonized in 1767.
45. J. France, *Les Femmes françaises pendant la guerre, 1870* (Limoges: Marc Barbou et cie., 1887), 89–90.
46. d'Erzerville, *Nos bonnes religieuses*, 43, gives her age as twenty-five and mentions only one condemned franc-tireur. Gustave Isambert's account in *Le Monde illustré* 15, no. 757 (14 October 1871), one of the first, claims that her nun's habit won her immediate respect due to the Catholicism of

the Bavarian regiment that occupied Chateaudun. Other versions of the story include L. Jablonski, *Les Femmes françaises à la guerre* (Paris: Henri Charles-Lavanauzelle, 1894), 126; Arnaud and Bonnette, *La Femme*, 80; and *Châteaudun pendant la guerre de 1870: Notice sur le dévouement de Soeur Jeanne de Chantal* (Bourges: Tardy-Pégelet, 1890). According to Sister Jeanne de Chantal's obituary, published in *Revue historique de l'Ouest* 12, 1 (1896): 12, she was thirty-seven in 1870, not fifty or twenty-five.

47. Le Fort, *La Chirurgie militaire*, 230–31.
48. M. H. Darrow, "The Story of Franco-Prussian War Heroine Coralie Cahen and the French Red Cross, 1871–1914," *Proceedings of the Western Society for French History* 36 (2008): 167–80. Cahen published her own account, *Souvenirs de la guerre de 1870–1871: Conférence faite le 25 mai 1888 au siège de l'Association des Dames françaises* (Paris: Association des Dames françaises, [1888]). Cahen was so well publicized in this period that the British magazine *Nursing Record* (3 January 1899): 10–11 cited her case in comparison to the lack of credit given to nurses in Britain.
49. The exceptions are articles in the Jewish press that highlight Cahen's work in Jewish charities rather than her war experiences. See, for example, B. M., "Madame Coralie Cahen," *L'Univers israélite* 55, no. 13 (17 March 1899): 805–9.
50. Cahen, *Souvenirs*, 11, 15.
51. The nurse-heroine was not the only propaganda figure that 1914 borrowed from 1870; there was also the little French boy with a toy gun killed by the Germans. In the 1914 version he was executed by firing squad; in the 1870 tale he was spitted by an uhlan's lance. See C. Roetter, *The Art of Psychological Warfare, 1914–1945* (New York: Stein and Day, 1974), 44.
52. M. Levée, "Faibles femmes . . . Femmes héroïques," *Minerva* (26 December 1937). Other accounts give other versions of his remark, such as "I hope, for our sake, there are not more women like you in France." Ernest Jean Delahaye's 1910 painting of this confrontation was much reproduced.
53. S. Tison, "Traumatisme de guerre et commémorations: Comment Champenois et Sarthois sont-ils sortis de la guerre? (1870–1940)," *Guerres mondiales et conflits contemporains* 216 (October 2004): 25.
54. M. Grillet, "Un convoi de blessés (Janville 1870)," *La Revue du siècle, littéraire, artistique & scientifique* 3, no. 3 (1889): 1–3.
55. Cahen, *Souvenirs*, 9.
56. Ambert, *Gaulois et Germains*, 2, 387.
57. de Valdor, "Les Femmes décorées," 233–34; C. Métais, "Chapelle de l'Hôtel-Dieu," *Archives du diocèse de Chartres*, 2nd series, 4 (1900): 15.
58. Cahen, *Souvenirs*, 9.
59. R. Chrastil, "The French Red Cross, War Readiness and Civil Society, 1866–1914," *French Historical Studies* 31, no. 3 (Summer 2008): 455–59. According to Hutchinson, *Champions of Charity*, 202–76, beginning in the 1880s, nationalism superseded humanitarianism across the affiliates of the International Red Cross, in Japan, the US, and in Europe.
60. Romangy, "Soeur Julie," 16.
61. *Appletons' Annual Cyclopaedia and Register of Important Events* 5 (1880): 658–59; *Sadliers' Catholic Directory, Almanac and Clergy List Quarterly* (New York: D. and J. Sadlier and Co., 1881), 38.
62. J-B. Didierjean, "Le Comte Henri de Verthamon, un héros de Loigny," *Etudes religieuses, philosophiques, historiques et littéraires, . . . publiées par des Pères de la Compagnie de Jésus* 27, no. 51 (September–December 1890): 260–64; Métais, "Chapelle de l'Hôtel-Dieu," 15; P. Champion, *Guillaume de Flavy* (Paris: Honoré Champion, éditeur, 1906), 452–55.

63. d'Ezerville, *Nos bonnes religieuses*, 39.
64. A. de Valdor, "Les Femmes infirmières," *La Femme et la famille* 60, no. 3 (March 1892): 68–70. See also A. L. Du Preÿ, *Les Femmes de 1870* (Saint-Omer: J. Devey, 1874), 61–62, 567; and journalist Jules Claretie, cited in Turquan, *Les Femmes*, 200.
65. Chrastil, "The French Red Cross," 462. See Taithe, *Defeated Flesh*, 134–37, for the campaign to secularize French nursing during the Paris Commune. J. D. Ellis, *The Physician-Legislators of France: Medicine and Politics in the Early Third Republic 1870–1914* (Cambridge: Cambridge University Press, 1990), 165–69, discusses the debate over hospital secularization in the French legislature in the 1880s and 1890s. Schultheiss, *Bodies and Souls*, recounts the struggle in municipalities and hospitals over the issue.
66. M. Du Camp, "La Bienfaisance israélite à Paris," part 2, *Revue des deux mondes* 83, 2 (15 September 1887): 278.
67. Cahen, *Souvenirs*,12.
68. J. Normand, "Association des Dames françaises: Madame Coralie Cahen," *La Revue bleue* 26, no. 2 (12 January 1889): 60.
69. C. Clermont, *Souvenirs de parisiennes en temps de guerre* (Paris: Berger-Levrault, 1918), 203; J. Crémieux, *Croquis d'heures vécues, 1914–1919* (Fourmies: Imp. Bachy, 1934), 39; M. Léra, *Les Provinces françaises pendant la guerre* (Paris: Librairie académique, Perrin et cie., 1918), 8, originally published as a series of articles in *Correspondant* in 1916 and 1917.
70. Marquise de Foucault, *A Château at the Front*, trans. G. B. Ives (Boston: Houghton Mifflin Company, 1931), 19–23.
71. Thébaud, *La Femme*, 88.
72. F. Lejars, *Un Hôpital militaire à Paris pendant la guerre: Villemin 1914–1919* (Paris: Masson et cie., 1923), 97–104.
73. "Pour soigner les blessés militaires: Appel aux femmes," *Le Petit Parisien* (6 August 1914); there is a similar article in *Echo de Paris* on 11 August.
74. Archives nationales, Paris, F7 12937 and 12938. See, for example, the report from the Prefect of the Calvados of 16 August and that of the Prefect of Deux-Sèvres of 11 August. The Prefect of the Basse-Alpes on 9 August applauded the women, whether or not they were "qualified," who volunteered to go anywhere they were needed to nurse: "these valiant women who have offered their services to the Government."

2 "Beacons of Britishness"

British Nurses and Female Doctors as Prisoners of War

Angela K. Smith

> Then the storm burst. The Germans and the Austrians advanced from the north; the Bulgarians swept into Macedonia from the east. It was known that all available regiments had been sent north and that, relying on the Allies, the military authorities had left the southern portion of the Bulgarian frontier practically undefended. Thus there were the makings of panic and disaster on a colossal scale.[1]

So wrote Leila, Lady Paget, in her account of the invasion of Serbia, printed for private circulation some months after her return to England in 1916. As she would also go on to record, the Allies never came. The Allies, or more specifically the British and the French, did not regard Serbia as strategically important enough to risk troops; they had other priorities. When it was flooded by the Austrian, German, and Bulgarian armies in late 1915, the Serbian army, weakened after three years of warfare, had no chance at all of holding them off.[2] Tens of thousands fled, both soldiers and civilians, and among them, most of the British women who had been working in hospital and relief units for various organizations since the beginning of the war. Lady Paget's husband, Sir Ralph, was the Commissioner for British Relief Units in Serbia, and he personally undertook to ensure that all the staff got out; a significant proportion of these were women. Some headed for Salonika, a gateway held by the British. Others, like those attached to Mabel St Clair Stobart's Third Serbian Relief Unit, accompanied the fleeing armies across the mountains of Montenegro and Albania to the west. But some, mostly doctors and nurses, Lady Paget among them, refused to go anywhere at all. Their sense of duty and their adherence to a set of ideals they associated with their national identity was too strong. Despite the fact that the British army did not come to Serbia's aid, or perhaps because of it, the women who stayed behind to run their hospitals, who chose to be prisoners of war, turned to a sense of their "Britishness" both to protect their medical charges and to make their own personal stands against their captors. If they were the only Allies prepared to fight for Serbia, they were determined to make their presence felt.

Serbia presented the ideal theater of war for these independent British women's medical units. Their offers of help had gone unheeded by the officers of the Royal Army Medical Corps (RAMC), despite their many qualifications and extensive experience.[3] Women were not deemed capable of taking charge and running the units themselves. But British women, including Lady Paget, had taken hospital units to the Balkans during the recent wars there, so the Serbian military authorities took a different view. They had seen British nurses at work firsthand and so understood their value and welcomed them.[4] They were also in desperate need of medical staff and not in any position to adopt the prejudices of the RAMC. This put the women who chose to go to Serbia in a rather paradoxical position. On the one hand they were "doing their bit" for king and country. On the other, they had to do it with another king's army in another country because the value of their service was not immediately recognized by their own. This reflects the fact the Allies did not prioritize the war in Serbia in their strategic planning; there was a place for the women because the Allied authorities sent no military resources. Indeed, as Jane Marcus has argued:

> The "Balkanization" of British women doctors and nurses in Serbia and Russia may be seen as part of a larger historical repression of the Eastern Front in favor of the story of Western Europe in histories of the war. The Eastern Front is the female "other" of World War I.[5]

In Serbia, the women not only carried out their more traditional role of military nursing, but as the war progressed they were forced to take on additional roles. Faced with invading armies, many of these women determined to remain with their patients, despite the threat of capture and the danger of becoming prisoners of war. As they waited with the Serbian people for the Allies to come to their aid, they also found that they were assumed by the local population to represent their nation, despite the fact that the British government would never have sanctioned them as official representatives. It was a strange dilemma.

In this chapter, I will argue that these British women saw themselves as serving the British war cause, despite their location in an alien land. Although an ally, Serbia had a reputation for being a rather wild and savage territory and was culturally very different to their British home. Yet it was an innate sense of patriotism, a commitment to what they understood as their Britishness, which motivated the women to remain. I also suggest that it was the culture of imperialism in which these women had been raised that stimulated this patriotism, giving them a sense of duty that was deeply embedded in their sense of personal identity. Julia Bush has argued that "the British Empire was a subject of interest, and even a source of pride and enthusiasm, for a great many Edwardian women."[6] But it was more than this. Imperialism enabled these women to see themselves as beacons of Britishness in all foreign lands, and that duty extended to representing their country if there were no menfolk around to do it. But because they were working as nurses and doctors, this placed them in a complex position. As carers, their duty was to prioritize their sick and wounded, embodying an ideal of transnational humanitarianism. But as British women, representing their country in a war zone, they often needed to assert themselves in other ways, leading to a need for twin identities that did not always sit comfortably together.

Serbia was an ally partly by default. Many saw the Serbs as responsible for triggering the war in the first place, as it was a Serbian student who had effectively fired the first shot. The assassination of the Austrian heir to the throne and an old allegiance with Russia brought Serbia into the conflict on the Allied side. While the conquest of Serbia offered Germany a useful communication route with her Ottoman allies to the south, her defense was seen as less of a priority by the British, who had other important battles to fight in 1915 with the attack at Gallipoli, as well as on the western front. However, the British women based in Serbia knew only that they were working with an ally, embroiled as they were in the daily life of the country. Lady Paget's First Serbian Relief Unit at Skoplje had been set up in mid-November 1914. Throughout the winter of 1914–1915, they had seen little fighting, but instead had been on hand to provide medical support and nursing care during the shattering typhus epidemic that raged across the country until the late spring of 1915. It had been a difficult winter, as Flora Scott, matron of the Skoplje hospital, recalled:

> It was terrible. At times I felt so helpless I did not know where to go and what to do first, and I began to wonder whether it was really worth going on. We were short of clothes, water, food and fires. It was too awful to see these poor creatures suffering and in want, yet helpless to do or give. The cold was intense, and there were deep snows, yet I could only give each man one blanket. Many had not even shirts. Often I felt I must give in. Yet on going round their faces would light up, and they were so grateful for the slightest attention it repaid one for all one's work.[7]

The terrible winter led into a long and relatively quiet summer. But they must have had little idea of what was going on elsewhere in the war. As they waited for the war to find them, they expected that any attack on Serbia would be repelled by the Allies as a matter of course. When the expected invasion came in October 1915 they began to take in the new casualties of war. But there was no response from the Allies. The situation in Serbia reached a crisis level very quickly. As the invading armies advanced, Paget traveled to Salonika to try to impress upon the British and French generals stationed there that the situation facing her hospital was very urgent. But her pleas fell on deaf ears. It appeared that the Allies had no immediate plans to intervene. As she returned to her unit, Paget began to see firsthand the exodus of the Serbian people as they fled:

> The station [at Veles] was in great disorder, the platform being packed with refugees and wounded who had crawled from the battle-field, and

> before the train finally drew up wounded and unwounded alike tried to rush it, hanging on the roofs, the one idea of the crowd being escape no matter how. Little children were trampled under foot and others hurled by their parents over the heads of the affrighted crowds into the horse boxes where the sick and wounded soldiers huddled together. Willing hands were out stretched to catch these little ones but many were injured. The scene was horrible. Women were screaming, children crying, men shouting, and it was impossible to help them as the frenzied mob was too intent on fighting its way into the train to pay attention to us, and we tried in vain to make ourselves heard above the din.[8]

Although Paget's account is retrospective, she manages to convey the chaos of the retreat. It echoes events witnessed and recorded by British nurses at this desperate time, in which Serbian society was out of control and in panic. The failure of the nurses to make their voices heard in the chaos seems to be an ironic reflection of Paget's failed meeting with the Allied generals. Nobody was listening to her; their pleas for quiet, for order, for assistance, all fell on deaf ears. Her focus on the plight of children gives the account an added poignancy. It is clear from her account that she believes the weakest will suffer the most in a situation where nobody listens. This vulnerability reinforces her need to offer aid. However, when she returned to her hospital the situation was even worse. The decision had been taken to evacuate all British medical and nursing staff. Two hundred Austrian prisoners of war who had been doing vital work as orderlies were also removed. The walking wounded joined the throng. But the hospital was full to bursting point with wounded men who could not be moved, and the invaders were approaching.

Of all the Allies, Serbia was hit very hard by the First World War. John Keegan has argued that Serbia was:

> The worst proportionate sufferer . . . of whose pre-war population of five million, 125,000 were killed or died as soldiers, but another 650,000 civilians succumbed to privation and disease, making a total of 15 per cent of the population lost, compared with something between two and three per cent of the British, French and German populations.[9]

Although a Christian kingdom, which should align it to Britain and her Allies, Serbia had only recently won independence from the Ottoman Turks who had ruled there for centuries. Thus, as Paget herself noted, Eastern Europe, embodied by Serbia, had been "lost to Christendom" five hundred years earlier following defeat at the battle of Kosovo.[10] The country occupied a curious sort of middle ground, not quite Western but not quite "Oriental" either. The repeated wars of recent years, most particularly the Balkan Wars of 1912 and 1913, had earned Serbia a rather warlike reputation, which when blended with the Ottoman connections gave the country as a whole a marginal status, being not quite of Europe: other. As I have argued, this difference, or otherness, is echoed in Serbia's very different attitude to the involvement of women in warfare, welcoming the British women's hospital units that other nations rejected, endorsing Jane Marcus's hypothesis about the "Balkanization" of British female doctors and nurses. Having had very recent experience of war also encouraged Serbians to welcome the women's medical units. In return, the country inspired a fierce loyalty in the British women who worked there. Many went on to campaign on Serbia's behalf after her defeat. Others remained after the war to help the country rebuild.[11]

Like several British women in medical units, Paget decided to stay as a result of both the ready acceptance of her skills and her sense of loyalty to Serbia. Despite the best efforts of her husband to get all the British women out, she understood that if she, as an upper-class British civilian woman, retained command of the hospital it might offer the wounded Serbians some protection. And if she could save the hospital stores, she would be in a position to offer aid to the stricken town as well as to the soldiers; a well-equipped hospital was a bargaining tool in wartime. The Serbian generals agreed to her staying although all the other nurses were told to go; only male medical staff was allowed to stay on. Paget's nurses refused to comply and argued that if they stayed and continued to serve the Serbian people, they might alleviate some of the bad feeling caused by the failure of the Allies to step in. They won the argument, but their decision was not an easy one:

> It is impossible to give a clear account of the next two or three days, of the increasing nightmare of horror that descended upon Skoplje, sweeping us into alternative moods of feverish activity and sullen lassitude, as rumour after rumour held sway. Our nerves and tempers varied like a barometer before a typhoon, the unceasing rain chilled our bodies and souls, and mud plastered all and everything with ugliness and desolation.[12]

Paget's metaphor of the barometer before a typhoon suggests a woman used to travel. She had certainly spent time in the Far East at the time of her marriage, as Sir Ralph Paget was Extraordinary Envoy and Minister Plenipotentiary to Siam. She had also lived in Germany before he was given the same role for the Kingdom of Serbia. But nothing had prepared her for this situation of defeat. All evacuating staff left by 21 October 1915, and the Bulgarians marched in a day later.

Because the Allies failed to come to Serbia's aid, the relationship between the British women and the country grew even more complex. The British nurses, who already stood out from the crowd because they were so clearly Western European, came to represent, for the Serbian people, the Allies on whom they were so depending. They internalized this expectation of their duty as British women, explaining why some would not leave despite the grave danger they now faced. It is true that by October 1915 many of the British women working in Serbia were in flight, along with most of the army and a good proportion of the civilian population. But Lady Paget was not the only one to refuse to leave her wounded. The founder of the Scottish Women's Hospitals, Dr. Elsie Inglis, also refused to leave her post at Krushevatz, which was taken by the Germans in November 1915:

> The German occupation of Krushevatz was heralded in proper form by bombardment. The Serbs blew up the railway bridge, which attracted their fire and they threw bombs and several shells into the town. We felt that we had had our baptism of fire.
>
> . . . Their entry next morning, 7th November, was almost in the form of an anti-climax. We turned into the principal street to find a German regiment lined up there. The best of the Serbs had left, white flags were hanging out of most of the occupied houses, and Krushevatz was taken.[13]

Like Paget, Inglis and her contingent of nurses became prisoners of war. And like Paget, their writings reveal that they were very conscious of their Britishness in that time of crisis. The Scottish Women's Hospitals, led by Elsie Inglis and funded by the Women's Suffrage Movement, put medical units across Europe during the First World War. The first unit arrived in Serbia in December 1914 and also employed Austrian prisoners of war to supplement the all-female nursing staff. Other units followed. They arrived in the midst of the typhus epidemic, and they suffered a number of casualties among their nursing staff during those first few months.[14] It was a kind of baptism of fire for them, even though the war itself took a relative backseat to begin with. No one could claim, therefore, that the nurses did not fully understand the dangers they faced and the possible consequences. Inglis knew exactly what she was doing when she opted to remain with her patients as the invasion began:

> It seemed to some of us impossible to leave her [Serbia] in her hour of catastrophe. We had come out to help, and now that help was most needed it was our clear duty to stand by. Sir Ralph Paget gave his consent to those staying who wished to. It was the good fortune of some of us that we were able to work for Serbs in a Serbian hospital as long as there were Serbs to work for. Others of us, who desired the same lot, were fated to spend dreary weeks as prisoners in Austria.[15]

When Inglis subsequently wrote about her time in Serbia, she took care to record the history of her intervention from a Serbian point of view. It is thus very clear that the bond established between the women and their Serbian allies was extremely strong. Inglis does not concern herself with the absent British, but with doing all she can to alleviate suffering in the face of that absence.

Other women, while agreeing to evacuation, also manifested a sense of loyalty to Serbia and a reluctance to leave the country to its fate. The unit of the Scottish Women's Hospitals under the control of Dr. Alice Hutchison, for example, was evacuated from Valjevo; however, moving them was not easy. Hutchison refused to leave anything behind to fall into enemy hands, but the nurses had only oxcarts as a means of transportation. The slow trek with all their equipment meant that they did not move fast enough to outrun the armies and were still in the town of Vrinjatcha Bania when it fell to the Austrians on 10 November 1915. They were only fifty miles away from their colleagues, Inglis's unit in Krushevatz, but all lines of communication were severed. Making use of both her nationality and her civilian status, Hutchison was quite determined to stand up to her captors. When the Austrian army commandeered all her hospital equipment before sending her on to Krushevatz, she refused to give it up without a receipt, insisting that after the war the Austrian government would be required to pay for it all under the terms of the Geneva Convention. Hutchison thereby made a point of ensuring that she understood her rights as a civilian in the arena of war, and she demanded that her captors adhere to those rights.

Hutchison's attitude, along with the responses of Paget, Inglis, and their nurses, was clearly influenced by the extent to which she confidently assumed and projected her identity as a British woman of high social status. These socially elite and highly educated women were products of a particular imperial kind of European culture that, as Edward Said has noted, "gained in strength and identity by setting itself off against the Orient as a sort of surrogate and even underground self."[16] And although Serbia was not the "Orient" in the accepted sense, it was alien enough in the setting of the First World War to inspire this kind of imperial confidence. As Julia Bush has argued, despite the primarily patriarchal nature of "Empire," "The spiritual creed of Empire was as attractive to many British women as it was to their male counterparts. It was an improving, self-reinforcing faith, designed to assert national vigor in an increasingly competitive world, but ultimately dependent on the personal qualities of the individual."[17] The "personal qualities of the individual" can be seen at work in each of these women as they draw on their upper-class status to assert their authority over their captors. Bush also suggests that "intrinsic to the imperial outlook was a self-definition of the British (often, interchangeably, 'Englishmen') as a peculiarly gifted race with an insatiable need to exert their colonizing genius for the benefit of less fortunate others."[18] Although there is no sense that these women were "colonizing" Serbia (despite the fact that many stayed on after the war), there is nonetheless something of this imperial benevolence in their determination to help the less fortunate, less developed, and substantially "different" Serbian people. Said comments, further, on the importance of "the idea of European identity as a superior one in comparison with all the non-European peoples and cultures" and on "the hegemony of European ideas about the Orient, themselves reiterating European superiority over Oriental backwardness."[19] Serbia, lost, in Paget's words, to Christendom for five hundred years, was in many ways non-European. As the invaders sweep in, the women began to see themselves as the protectors of their "Oriental" Serbian charges, bolstered by that innate sense of Imperial superiority. Of course, some of the invaders were Western Europeans, too, but they were not British and were demonized as "barbarian," uncivilized, and brutal. This was one of the reasons behind the women's strong sense of self-righteousness, which enabled them to stand up for their rights and the rights of their patients. For women like Hutchison, the mere fact that the enemy troops were prepared to take civilian nurses prisoner indicated the level of their barbarity and transgression of "civilized" wartime codes of behavior. The existing treaties of the Geneva Conventions (1864 and 1906), together with the stipulations of the Hague Conventions (1899 and 1907), made it clear how civilians should be treated in a war situation, and Hutchison was well aware of this.[20] These female doctors and nurses, products of an imperial society, were thereby convinced that "right" was on their side; they must have been quite a daunting prospect for their captors.

For the rest of 1915, the British women prisoners survived as best they could and attempted to negotiate with their captors. They all determinedly held on to their sense of Britishness, and wherever they could they used it as a kind of beacon as they continued to give aid to the other victims of the invasion. Initially, after the Bulgarians had taken Skoplje, Paget noted: "The English were now questioned more closely as to why the Allies so long delayed their coming. In those evil days old Serbian friends, with whom we had faced death all through the typhus-scourge of the previous winter, turned away from us, hardly knowing whether we were friends or foes."[21] In order to combat this kind of thinking, the nurses worked hard to demonstrate British goodwill. They were faced with a disturbing paradox, which may be described by adopting Homi Bhabha's phrase the "impossible unity of nation as symbolic force."[22] The women were seen by many as the physical embodiment of Britain and, therefore, by extension, of the Allies. They were perceived as representing the "unity" of the British nation and so needed to carry the full symbolic weight of the Allies as they went about their daily tasks. However, they were not formal representatives in any way, however much their imperial upbringing may have instilled the importance of their nationality in them. As Bhabha argues is always the case with imperial writing, they manifest an awareness that they were not really part of a "united nation"; they, too, were waiting for Allies who would never come. Thus, while they carried out the role of benevolent imperial ladies, distributing aid to the local residents, most of whom had been left with nothing, at the same time Paget used her British citizenship and civilian status to ensure that the unit received good treatment and was not detained for too long. It was one thing to make a stand, to remain, and to ensure that their patients were not ill-treated, but ultimately as British medical women they should not be kept long as prisoners of war. By the end of 1915 the women were confident that they had done all they could:

> I pointed out quite clearly to [the Bulgarian chief medical officer] . . . that we might have escaped, but had chosen to stay and be made prisoners rather than abandon our work. I explained that we were a unit supported by a public fund raised in England to help the Serbians, and that I should have to account both to my Government and my committee, as soon as I got home, for everything I had done. I said we were willing to give help to the wounded Bulgarians until they could make their own medical arrangements, but that I formally demanded as soon as it was practicable, to be sent home with my entire staff.[23]

Paget's tone here implies that sense of imperial superiority, no doubt endorsed by her status as an upper-class British woman. A "democratic" public fund, specifically English, supports this; they cannot let down the ordinary English people who have invested in them.[24] She draws on the higher authorities of the British government and her committee as evidence of the importance of their commitment. Surprisingly, the "committee" almost seems to carry more weight than the government, highlighting the importance of the notion of British women's imperial or benevolent societies in Paget's frame of reference. This situation brings out the real paradox of the twin roles performed by these medical women. On the one hand, they were doctors and nurses, dedicated above all things to the care of their wounded, Serbian and Bulgarian alike. On the other, as British women, envoys of the Allies, they needed to assert their patriotic, imperialist sense of superiority that would enable them to take the moral high ground with their enemies. The demand to be sent home places authority firmly back in the hands of the leader of the unit, not the invading soldiers, but it is not without its moral complications for their position as doctors and nurses.

Similar demands were made by the other captive women, but it appears that their value was as great to their captors as it had been to the Serbian army. At Krushavetz the Germans took over Inglis's hospital, forcing all the nurses to move to the Czar Lazar, the Serbian military hospital. This was meant to accommodate up to nine hundred patients, but the numbers rose to twelve hundred during the women's time there. In addition to this, the hospital was surrounded by thousands of prisoners of war being moved to Hungary, for whom they felt obliged to care.

> The existence of misery they led was indescribable, as was the filth amongst which they lived . . . The hospital itself possessed the most

> villainous sanitary appointments it has ever been my lot to behold. The glorious sunsets, the hills, all around the town picturesquely against the soft colouring of the sky . . . how incongruous it all was.[25]

With sanitation such a problem, typhus was a significant threat, but the nurses adapted a disinfection machine to heat water and managed to avoid the disease completely.[26] Clearly this was very important in altruistic terms, but equally it was necessary for the women to demonstrate their understanding of humanitarian treatment for all prisoners of war. Again, this understanding enabled them to occupy the moral high ground. In her discussion of POWs, Sibylle Scheipers has argued that "during the twentieth century, prisoners became an increasingly important aspect of war propaganda. Emphasizing one's own humane treatment of prisoners and condemning the opponent's treatment of prisoners was often intended to enhance the international reputation of a state."[27] While the women were busy ensuring that they did the absolute best for all patients no matter which side they were on, Elsie Inglis certainly had firsthand experience of this concern from the other point of view. When the Germans moved out in late November, handing the town over to the Austrians, they asked her to sign a document testifying to their good behavior. Despite being threatened and harassed, she refused. She was concerned that the propaganda value of such a document would be too great, particularly with regard to women prisoners. The 1915 execution of British nurse Edith Cavell, in Belgium, was still fresh in everyone's minds. The Germans had received a good deal of international criticism for this execution, despite the fact that Cavell had pleaded guilty to the charge of helping British and Belgian soldiers to escape occupied territory. Inglis was very conscious of this, and she was not prepared to do anything that might inadvertently improve the international reputations of her captors.

At the same time, the reluctance of Elsie Inglis is also understandable given the fact that the living conditions of the nurses were quite shocking. It is likely that Inglis felt that the Germans did not deserve her endorsement. Dr. Helen McDougall later wrote:

> Black sour bread—we might have sugar in coffee if we liked, but no sugar elsewhere—thin soup and bean mess, with limited rough meat at lunch, and as often as not the bean mess again at night. . . . There was no milk, no eggs, nothing at all of the lighter sort. It may sound all right to those who have never tried it, but for myself the black bread was sometime scarcely eatable, yet from experience I knew it was better than none.[28]

Nothing in their medical training had prepared the women for privations of this sort, just as nothing had prepared them for imprisonment. Alice Hutchison noted:

> I came across Dr. Inglis and her Unit. If I had up till then felt that we in no way merited the title of "the heroic band of women," I came away from Dr. Inglis' hospital feeling that they *had* earned it. Picture over twenty people—including the head of the hospital—dining and sleeping and eating and washing in one room; picture all their equipment gone, and them looking after Serbs in the best way they could in hospital corridors. They were however, wearing no air of martyrdom.[29]

Hutchison is very aware of the way the women may be perceived from the outside, that their being prisoners of war might earn them a particular reputation. While determined not to accept any such accolade for herself, as this is a kind of heroism usually reserved for male combatants and she is clearly uncomfortable about it from her position as a civilian woman, Hutchison acknowledges that Inglis and her nurses really have earned this status of martyr-heroine. However, it is also clear that the women have internalized and modeled the behaviors of the British imperial heroine here, as they continued to carry out their hospital work under extreme conditions. Again, this is reflective of notions of the heroism of work "against the odds" in the British Empire. As Bush puts it, "duty and responsibility, interest and honour impelled the British to sustain their imperial burden,"[30] and for decades British men and women had attempted to reproduce the heroic qualities associated with this duty.

While the nurses tended the wounded in Krushavetz and Paget and her company worked to restore the tarnished British image in Skoplje, Alice Hutchison's unit was forced to join the thousands of prisoners of war being herded toward Hungary. Their encounter with Inglis took place after they had been removed from Vrinjatcha Bania. A brief stopover in Krushavetz showed them what they might expect on their own journey. When they reached their destination, Kevevara, thirty-two of them were accommodated in two rooms. They were held there for five weeks, but unlike the women in other locations they were not given any work, so for them the monotony was as great a trial as the black bread. Days were spent waiting to be restored to them. Hutchison continued to argue that as a civilian woman, it was a breach of the Geneva Convention for her to be held as a prisoner of war at all, but for weeks her argument fell on deaf ears.

In December there was an outbreak of cholera among the Serbian prisoners, and Hutchison was instructed to take charge. She remembered the directives of the Hague Conventions relating to prisoners of war and work: "They could be employed in work, so long as it was not related to war operations, nor should it be exhausting or humiliating."[31] Nursing the sick Serbian prisoners, their Allies, did not count as inappropriate war work as such, but exposing themselves to the acute danger of sickness or death did contravene the dictates of the Conventions. She drew on her authority as an educated British civilian woman and refused to allow her nurses to work unless they were all first vaccinated against the disease. "Then came a torrent of the most uncontrolled abuse and threats that I have ever been subjected to—incarceration to the end of the war, starvation, treatment as ordinary prisoner, &c."[32] But Hutchison stood firm, and the nurses were never forced to work in the cholera hospital. It was another moral victory for the women prisoners.

Christmas found all the units still in captivity. A determination to celebrate it regardless of their circumstances provided Hutchison's unit with a sense of patriotism that helped to carry them through. In effect, celebrating Christmas became a symbol of their Britishness, particularly as their Christmas did not fall in line with the Serbian orthodox calendar. Hutchison notes that their guards, who would have shared their festive season, had become quite friendly by Christmas Day, and they were able to celebrate far better than they had expected:

> On Christmas Day we had quite a jolly time, with a Christmas tree and a first-rate dinner. We went out and got some live geese from the market, which were killed and cooked, and we had all kinds of cakes, and even butter. . . . In the evening we sang carols and drank toasts. We even ventured for the first time to sing "God Save the King" under our breath. After this we sang it every night, and it cheered us up wonderfully.[33]

In comparison with the usual diet of black bread, this seems quite luxurious. However, what is most significant here is the singing of the national anthem, the reclaiming and celebration of national identity. This freedom, gained through the occasion, becomes a part of their daily ritual; an assertion of their nationhood, the British Empire, and, by implication, their superiority. Their captors are not to be allowed to forget their Britishness. This refusal to forget who they are unites all these women, and it helps them to face the extraordinary challenges to their identities both personal and national.

Their assertion of a "morally superior" imperial brand of British womanhood appears to have worked. With the dawning of 1916, the German, Austrian, and Bulgarian armies determined to rid themselves of the British women prisoners in their midst. Lady Paget had enjoyed the patronage of Eleanora, the queen of the Bulgarians, with whom she had worked in the Balkan Wars of 1912 and 1913. The queen's personal history of war nursing and these previous associations with British medical women during the Balkan Wars made her very sympathetic to the work of the various hospitals.[34] Although there is no direct evidence to suggest that this was why Paget's unit was released, the queen may have had some influence. Paget had also adopted a policy of gentle negotiation with her captors and later believed that this, in the end, led to a smoother passage home for her party. She also disassociated herself publicly from anyone she defined as "pro-Serbian" during their return journey, because she thought any such connection would lead to their being detained for the duration of the war. She endeavored to remain as neutral as possible, foregrounding her medical role and its intersection with her British one throughout the process of her release, adopting only an impression of British calm, reserve, and, above all, control throughout.

The first Serbian Relief Unit left Skoplje on 17 February 1916:

> It was not very easy to leave the hospital, though it held for us the memory of so much pain and hard work. It had been brought forth in sorrow, when typhus held the land in its grip. It had risen up out of the filth and disease in which we found it, by the labours of a few, till by degrees it had become one of the best-equipped hospitals in Serbia . . . I had not realised till the moment came to leave how much I had hoped to hand it back to the Serbians. Never had the mountains looked more serene or more beautiful than in that early morning light, but it was a sad leave we took of the poor Serbian captives, and tears rolled down the faces of our faithful Austrians.[35]

Imperial benevolence appears to play its part here. The "poor Serbian captives" and the "faithful Austrians" (prisoners of war previously captured by the Serbians who had been working as orderlies) are still presented as needing the protection of the women and by proxy, of the Allies. But as Allies, they have failed their charges, leaving them in the hands of their captors. It was to be a long trip home. The group was detained further in Sofia for four weeks. Paget refused to travel home through Germany, and their progress was hampered by continual reports from German officials that they were all spies. When the Swiss border was closed to them, they were forced to travel home via Russia and did not arrive in London until 3 April 1916. Despite her determination to uphold her Britishness and to represent the absent Allies, Paget and her nurses were criticized on their return for getting on too well with the Bulgarian queen. Perhaps because of her previous connection to the queen, it had been inaccurately reported that they had been her guests in Sofia, whereas, in fact, they were accommodated by the Bulgarian Red Cross. Here again is the paradox, Bhabha's "impossible unity of nation as symbolic force." The women had symbolically embodied Britain and the Allies and had put themselves at great personal risk in order to uphold the international reputation of their nation. Yet the nation, in its most formal sense, seemed blind to this endeavor. Because the women could be deemed to have transgressed in their dealing with the enemy queen, the nation distanced itself from them. Sadly this is fairly representative of the British attitude more generally to hospital and relief work in Serbia, much of it undertaken by women. At home they went unappreciated, even criticized for their efforts. Unlike the trained and volunteer nurses who went to other fronts, they had not been sanctioned and were treated with suspicion. The Serbians, however, awarded Lady Paget the Order of Saint Sava, First Class. For them, her twin roles both deserved formal recognition.

Elsie Inglis's unit left Krushavetz on 9 February 1916. They were escorted to neutral Switzerland by an armed Austrian guard with fixed bayonets. "Great care was taken that we should not communicate with any one *en route*."[36] Inglis, perhaps, had appeared to her captors to be a little more recalcitrant or threatening. They were handed over to the American embassy in Vienna and from there received safe passage home. Having spent nearly four months waiting to leave Serbia, Inglis had not yet given up hope of further help for the Serbians she had left behind: "When we reached Zurich and found everything much the same as when we disappeared into the silence, our hearts were sick for the people we left behind us still waiting and trusting."[37] "The silence" may be a strange way to describe a war zone, but it gives an accurate impression of that zone in the eyes of the British and French military. Eva Shaw McClaren suggests that the experience of leaving Serbia was deeply traumatic for Inglis: "those who know her best feel that it was here, going in spirit with her beloved Serbs through their time of extremest woe, that Dr. Inglis' 'heart broke' and the 'beginning of the end' came upon her."[38] Later that year, Elsie Inglis led another unit of the Scottish Women's Hospitals to Russia, and she died of cancer shortly after her return home on 26 November 1917. In death, however, Inglis did receive the recognition of her homeland. Her funeral in Edinburgh was attended by thousands and was followed by the founding of the Elsie Inglis Memorial Hospital in the city, while another was also founded in Belgrade.

Throughout her captivity, Alice Hutchison secretly preserved the unit's Union Jack flag. When they left Budapest for Vienna on 4 February 1916, she wound it around her body underneath her clothes for safekeeping, determined not to see it trampled and insulted. As their train passed over the Swiss border, the unit produced the flag waving it from the train windows in triumph, shouting "God Save the King." They had retained, or perhaps reinforced, their sense of Britishness in the face of oppression and were prepared to shout about it to the world. Thus their British identity remained dominant despite their adoption of a more transitional humanitarian identity as nurses. It was, however, the combination of these twin strands that enabled them to prevail and secure their release while continuing to give as much support to their Allies as possible.[39]

The operations of British women in Serbia in the First World War were an extraordinary phenomenon. Serbia presented British women with a theater of war in which they could be active, could "do their bit," when the British government had made it clear that independent women on active service, even medical women, were largely undesirable. It was a paradoxical situation from the start. The culture of empire, and imperial sensibility, internalized since childhood, fed these women's desire to play a part in the war that threatened the whole of society, and indeed, the empire itself. This unquestioning adoption of a particular brand of "Britishness" gave them the confidence to face up to and overcome dangers, retaining and upholding their national identity despite being isolated by their own countrymen and having to watch the nation to which they had committed themselves in service fall into despair and defeat. Despite its hardships, imprisonment in Serbia allowed these women to demonstrate their strength and skills, and, for many, being able to stay on and support Serbia as it fell must have made up, in some small way, for the failings of a male military machine that regarded a small ally as being not important enough to save. It also offered them the chance to explore and gain new confidence in their identities while prisoners of war. They were both Edwardian women and medics; they had used the experiences of both these roles to take control of their situation, understanding themselves as "beacons of Britishness" throughout their captivity.

NOTES

1. Lady L. Paget, *With Our Serbian Allies: Second Report* (printed for private circulation: 1916), 9, Imperial War Museum, 34602.
2. The Serbians had been at war with the Ottoman Empire in the two Balkan Wars of 1912–1913.
3. Dr. Elsie Inglis of the Scottish Women's Hospitals was famously told "to go home and keep quiet" when she offered her medical unit to the War Office. See R. Strachey, *The Cause* (London: Virago, 1978 [1928]), 338.
4. Mabel St Clair Stobart took the Women's Sick and Wounded Convoy Corps to Bulgaria in 1912. See A. K. Smith, "The Woman Who Dared: Major Mabel St. Clair Stobart," in *The Women's Movement in Wartime: International Perspectives 1914–19*, ed. A. S. Fell and I. Sharp (Basingstoke: Palgrave, 2007), 158–174. Lady Paget also worked closely with the Queen of Bulgaria.
5. J. Marcus, "Corpus/Corps/Corpse: Writing the Body in/at War," in *Arms and the Woman: War, Gender and Literary Representation*, ed. H. M. Cooper, A. A. Munich, and S. M. Squier (Chapel Hill: University of North Carolina Press, 1989), 135.
6. J. Bush, *Edwardian Ladies and Imperial Power* (London: University of Leicester Press, 2000), 16.
7. F. Scott, The Papers of Miss Flora Scott, Matron of the Sixth Military Reserve Hospital, Skoplje, Imperial War Musem, Documents 6977.
8. Paget, *With Our Serbian Allies*, 12.
9. J. Keegan, *The First World War* (London: Pimlico, 1999), 7.
10. Paget, *With Our Serbian Allies*, 22.
11. For example, after the war Dr. Katherine Macphail of the Scottish Women's Hospitals opened a hospital for tubercular children first on the Dalmation coast, then moving north of Belgrade, and remained there until the Second World War. Evelina Haverfield, the administrator of the Scottish Women's Hospitals, did likewise at Bajina Basta until her death in 1920. See M. Krippner, *The Quality of Mercy* (London: David and Charles, 1980).
12. Paget, *With Our Serbian Allies*, 19–20.
13. E. Inglis, "The Tragedy of Serbia," *Englishwoman* 30 (1916): 166.
14. See L. Leneman, *In the Service of Life: The Story of Elsie Inglis and the Scottish Women's Hospitals* (Edinburgh: Mercat Press, 1994), 20–21.

15. E. Inglis, "The Tragedy of Serbia," in *Women's Writing of the First World War: An Anthology*, ed. A. K. Smith (Manchester: Manchester University Press, 2000), 270.
16. E. W. Said, *Orientalism* (London: Penguin, 2003), 3.
17. Bush, *Edwardian Ladies*, 2.
18. Ibid., 1.
19. Said, *Orientalism*, 7.
20. For further information, see A. R. Kramer, "Prisoners in the First World War," in *Prisoners in War*, ed. S. Scheipers (Oxford: Oxford University Press, 2010), 76–77.
21. Paget, *With Our Serbian Allies*, 20.
22. H. K. Bhabha, *Nation and Narration* (London: Routledge, 1990), 1.
23. Paget, *With Our Serbian Allies*, 36–37.
24. As Bush notes, "Intrinsic to the imperial outlook was a self-definition of the British (often, inter-changeably, 'Englishmen')" (Bush, *Edwardian Ladies*, 1).
25. Dr. Helen McDougall, quoted in Leneman, *In the Service of Life*, 42.
26. For more details see Leneman, *In the Service of Life*, 42–43.
27. S. Scheipers, *Prisoners in War* (Oxford: Oxford University Press, 2010), 8.
28. Helen McDougal from an article published in *The Instructor: Journal for the Children of the Free Church in Scotland* (April 1917), quoted in Leneman, *In the Service of Life*, 42–43.
29. Alice Hutchison, quoted in E. Shaw McLaren, *A History of the Scottish Women's Hospitals* (London: Hodder and Stoughton, 1919), 164.
30. Bush, *Edwardian Ladies*, 1–2.
31. Kramer, "Prisoners in the First World War," 76.
32. Hutchison, quoted in Leneman, *In the Service of Life*, 44–45.
33. Alice Hutchison, quoted in E. Shaw McClaren, *A History of the Scottish Women's Hospitals* (London: Hodder and Stoughton, 1919), 164.
34. Eleanora, queen of the Bulgarians, had worked with Mabel St Clair Stobart and her field hospital units, who had participated in the Balkan War of 1912.
35. Paget, *With Our Serbian Allies*, 93.
36. E. Inglis, "The Tragedy of Serbia,", *Englishwoman* 30 (1916), 171.
37. Ibid.
38. McClaren, *A History*, 172.
39. Dr. Hutchison continued to serve with the Scottish Women's Hospitals until the end of the war. After the war she devoted herself to children's medicine, working in a number of hospitals, including Great Ormond Street.

3 "I Begin to Feel as a Normal Being Should, in Spite of the Blood and Anguish in Which I Move"

American Women's First World War Nursing Memoirs

Jane Potter

INTRODUCTION: THE AMERICAN MISSION

> Our object now, as then, is to vindicate the principles of peace and the justice in the life of the world as against selfish and autocratic power and to set up amongst the really free and self-governed peoples of the world such a concert of purpose and of action as will henceforth insure the observance of those principles. . . . The world must be made safe for democracy. Its peace must be planted upon the tested foundations of political liberty. We have no selfish ends to serve. We desire no conquest, no dominion. We seek no indemnities for ourselves, no material compensation for the sacrifices we shall freely make. We are but one of the champions of the rights of mankind.
>
> (Address of the president of the United States delivered at a joint session of the two houses of Congress, 2 April 1917[1])

The United States occupied a unique position between 1914 and 1918: first as a seemingly detached spectator and second as a crusading participant. Yet it is this supreme confidence in the country's mission "to vindicate the principles of peace and the justice in the life of the world as against selfish and autocratic power" (we hear resonances today[2]) that marks the particularly American response to the "war to end all war." Naive in its assuredness, evangelical in its outlook, the sense of mission is reflected in the writings of American noncombatant witnesses, particularly nurses. Now largely forgotten, a significant corpus of writing exists, published and unpublished. Previous scholarly studies have tended to focus on a limited number of what may be considered canonical works, such as Mary Borden's *The Forbidden Zone* (1929) and Ellen La Motte's *The Backwash of War* (1916), both of which are considered elsewhere in this volume. This chapter, however, seeks to illuminate less well-known writings, by less famous women. Published accounts and letters home to family served to enlighten a distant American public—"distant" both in geography and in mind.[3] Published memoirs in particular sought to encourage financial support for various aid associations and, above all, to bear witness to the suffering of the fighting men. Their role as pro-war, pro-Allies propaganda should also not be underestimated. Indeed, they formed part of the unofficial means by which the country became convinced of the need for its involvement in this European conflict.[4] This chapter will explore how, despite all the self-conscious certainty that the US is the beacon of light for the world, these memoirs and letters are decidedly more contradictory and multifaceted than a first glance at the assured exterior would indicate.

American nurses in the First World War found themselves confronting multiple paradoxes or double binds, the "unresolvable sequence of experiences" and messages that "come to be an habitual expectation."[5] Firstly, they experienced the double bind affecting all medical personnel in wartime: the imperative to heal the men in their care set against the military imperative to return those same men to the fighting. Secondly, they negotiated a double bind unique to them as Americans, one distinguished by moral outrage and detachment on the one hand (America as "a city on a hill") and a moral investment and active participation on the other (America as a world police, the armed "champions of mankind"). The shifting nature of American nurses' position with regard to their country's involvement added a further level of paradox: before April 1917, these volunteers were in the war, but not of it—they were not citizens of an official combatant nation. They could and did judge the conflict in multiple ways that varied from the feeling of superiority that such chaos was not of their making to a disdain for the inaction of their American government. After April 1917 they were faced with the unsettling reality that the terrible suffering of the men—American troops in particular—was the result of recruitment efforts in which they themselves were complicit. Nursing and other memoirs published before the US joined the Allies attempted to coerce, if not to shame, a desultory citizenry into action, while those published after aimed to strengthen the resolve of a nation that, through its president, claimed to seek "no conquest, no dominion." The nurses' sense of their political and national selves, filtered down through their writing, was the product of an education that "assigned a redemptive role to the United States, fighting evil to create a new international order."[6] Thus, while they share many characteristics with those of British nurses—graphic descriptions of wounds; the feelings of helplessness buoyed by a sense of duty; the devotion to the patients in their care; and, in the aftermath, a sense of loss, isolation, and sadness—the memoirs considered here are distinctly American, their authors viewing themselves (whatever their age) as the offspring of a new and bright nation, distinct from the Old World, whose redemptive mission made them witnesses to and actors in a global conflict.

THE SPECTACLE OF THE EUROPEAN WAR

In 1914 America was able to view the situation in Europe from a distance, but even so it was not immune to the arguments for and against its participation in this foreign conflict, and women played a key role in both sides of the debate. Many were eager for the US to do its part. War-tourists, made up largely of "lady novelists," made their way to Europe from August 1914 onward. Their stated purpose was to muster US financial support for the Allied war effort, and they did so by employing the highly charged language and purple prose of their fiction, reinforcing "the romance of war," despite distressing details. The undeclared, implicit perk of such fact-finding missions was their opportunity for exciting adventure (interestingly, all of these women were middle-aged or elderly). Stanley Cooperman described them as seeing "American troops as Boy Scouts out on a field trip."[7] Margaret Higonnet has noted how Ellen La Motte, in her first essay about her experiences, "criticizes dilettantes who are contributing token time and effort to hospital tasks. . . . Society girls who are gathering 'experiences which will tell well in next year's ballroom.'"[8] Among the dilettantes might be Mary Roberts Rinehart, whose *Kings, Queens and Pawns* was published in 1915, as was Edith Wharton's *Fighting France* and Mildred Aldrich's *A Hilltop on the Marne.*[9] Seemingly in their defense (though perhaps adding to the criticism), Gertrude Atherton, in her memoir *Life in the War Zone* (1916), declared that:

> a certain type of smug American, who, without experience or imagination, has refused to believe in the attendant horrors of war, should be encouraged to visit these deliberately wrecked towns and hear at first hand far worse stories than even Lord Bryce has printed. . . . Let these self-righteous citizens, who have grown fat on the European war, take a motor trip through the ruined district a year hence and spend an hour or two with the survivors.[10]

This quotation not only demonstrates the way in which British propaganda (in particular, the Bryce Report on Alleged German Atrocities[11]) was widely circulated, but Atherton puts herself in a privileged position by adding her evidence. She tries to bring home the horrors of war, but her call to "take a motor trip" no doubt would have irritated the military men who wanted to keep such spectators out of the war zone.

One popular novelist who did more than take a motor trip was Marie van Vorst. Her memoir *War Letters of an American Woman* (1916) details her struggles to become and her experiences as a frontline nurse with the American Ambulance in France.[12] She first has to overcome the prejudice of women like Mrs. Vanderbilt, who believed van Vorst was only taking Red Cross exams for the excitement. Placed in distressing and difficult situations "to see what I could stand, or how soon she could get rid of me," van Vorst, to her "tremendous surprise," "found myself able to bear a very great deal." She assists in "two of the dressings without feeling the slightest atom of nausea, and carried away pile after pile of that loathsome, infected linen . . . several times I felt, not like fainting, but like weeping my heart out."[13] But she is candid about the self-control and fortitude her nursing requires and admits to a change of attitude to those she too had previously mocked:

> I shall never forget the courage it took to take the safety-pins out of a gangrened wound for the first time: it wasn't pleasant. It's all very well to laugh at amateur nurses, and if you will recall one of my letters, written in London during the times of my Red Cross examinations, you will see that I laughed first and with you. But that is all changed. The auxiliaries and the amateurs at the American Ambulance have done perfectly marvelous work. Those ladies gifted first with intelligence and tenderness, common sense and dignity, are now difficult to distinguish—some of them—from the professionals; and even as far as the battle line, lying so red and so trampled in Belgium, they have done superb work.[14]

Such memoirs not only lauded the efforts of American women "gifted . . . with intelligence and tenderness, common sense and dignity," but added to the public fascination with events overseas, some of which led to organized societies. The women's section of the Navy League was founded in 1915 and other pseudo-military organizations followed. Indeed, as Erika Kuhlman has shown, some progressive pacifists from groups such as the World Peace Foundation, the American Union against Militarism, and even the Women's Peace Party accepted the idea of "reasonable preparedness."[15] While hundreds of women joined the "Mass Meeting for Peace" on 2 April 1917, the day the US declared war on Germany, and while others continued to resist any involvement in voluntary relief work or paid employment in war industries, many feminists in particular faced the difficult decision to support the government once it pledged the country to the Allies.

"NOBODY IS A SPECTATOR": AMERICA ENTERS THE WAR

President Wilson in his address to "his fellow countrymen" in April 1917 declared that "the supreme test of our nation has come. We must all speak, act and serve together!"[16] Up until this moment, Margaret Deland argued that "American knowledge of what war means had been Academic." Now "everybody is in the Cast of the Terrible Show—nobody is a Spectator."[17] Deland is particularly impressed with what she calls the "exodus of American girls" and "the passionate desire on the part of the women of one people to go to the help of the men of another people." Contrary to La Motte's criticism, Deland wonders whether "any other nation . . . if we were at war, would send its girls across to serve us?" But in keeping with this supreme confidence in American ideals she asserts:

> I am inclined to think that this special expression of [Altruism], which has started a little army of girls over to France, could not have happened anywhere but in the United States, where fathers and mothers have so very little to say as to the behavior of their daughters . . . they cannot

> hold their girls back from the gray sea, where heaven only knows what may meet them![18]

The liberality of parenting, particularly in relation to girls, is expressed as something quintessentially American, slightly bohemian even, but put to good use when challenged for the greater good. These daughters were not held back, for "heaven knows what might meet them" was part of the attraction. The neutrality agreement did not forbid noncombatant involvement or recruitment, "so Americans began to flood the volunteer movement."[19] One hundred and fifty nurses and forty-five surgeons were sent to France by the American Red Cross in the first five months of the war. Harvard University sent 110 skilled, experienced doctors and nurses to a new camp hospital in July 1915 and many individuals from American universities joined the three ambulance corps services overseas.[20]

Events such as the execution of Edith Cavell in 1915 galvanized American outrage. In an effort to memorialize this victim of German barbarity, a committee in Boston was formed to appoint a special "Edith Cavell Memorial Nurse" to serve with the British army in France. Forty-one-year-old Alice Fitzgerald, who had been working for most of her life to promote her profession, was appointed. On 19 February 1916, she sailed for England and was eventually attached to the Queen Alexandra's Imperial Military Nursing Service at Boulogne. Fitzgerald felt particularly duty-bound as an American to show she could work hard and withstand the hellish conditions, especially when she was transferred to a Casualty Clearing Station. Her success is attested to by Helen Fraser, an official of the War Savings Committee of the British Treasury, who gave a series of lectures to women's colleges in the US on various topics related to the war. These lectures, later published as *Women and War Work* in 1917, argued that the appointment "shows the unity of your feeling and ours on that tragic execution." The dust jacket of the volume declares that Fraser is "anxious to do all in her power to help American women, passing from a peace to a war basis." On the subject of medical help, the British woman extols the involvement of her American sisters:

> With America our link has always been very great and all the help, and gifts, and service America gave us before it entered the war, have been very precious to us. American women have given Hospitals and ambulances and everything possible in the way of succour and of service, and have died with our women in nursing service, as the men have in our ranks . . . the work of all the American nurses we have had helping us is another link in the great chain.[21]

The link in the great chain was further strengthened with the first mobilization of nurses in June 1917 stationed at the US Quarantine Hospital, Island No. 3, Ellis Island, New York. A further 250 nurses from US Army

General Hospital No. 1, Williamsbridge, New York City, were mobilized on 8 September 1917, followed by others from stations at Hoboken, New Jersey, and the Colony Club, Madison Avenue, New York City. In her history of the Army Nurse Corps, Julia Stimson pointedly noted that "no member of the Army Nurse Corps, either regular or reserve, was assigned to overseas service against her will."[22]

Charles F. Thwing praised the courage and dedication of American college women, in particular, asserting that their service "at home and abroad":

> proves that their hearts have the same patriotic beat as the hearts of their brothers . . . they are the saviors of their race quite as truly as their fathers, brothers, husbands and children. . . . In conditions demanding heroism quite as great and endurance quite as severe, without resulting decorations of war crosses or orders of merit, they have proved themselves to be the worthiest.[23]

Such high-minded language is resonant of that used by the novelists/war-tourists, and it stands in marked contrast to the more matter-of-fact style (though it is not without a certain lyricism) of nurses whose memoirs are considered in this chapter.

The first American nurse to die in France was Amabel Scharff Roberts. Educated at Columbia University, she served at Base Hospital Number 2 with the Presbyterian Hospital, where she died in January 1918 having contracted blood poisoning. Three army nurses were awarded the Citation Star for gallantry in action: Jane I. Rignel, Linnie Leckrone, and Irene Robar. Rignel was Chief Nurse of Mobile Hospital No. 2, attached to the Forty-Second Division, at Bussy-le-Château, when she continued to treat the wounded under heavy enemy fire. One nurse from the same unit recalled how:

> stretcher after stretcher was brought in until it seemed as if there were no more beds to hold them. They came in filth and grime—torn, weak, exhausted masses of tortured flesh and broken bones, their faces pale and ghastly with the agony of their terrible ordeal . . . No sooner had we ministered to one than another was at hand . . . but through it all splendid bits of heroism that brought a catch to the throat. All the work was done under continuous shell fire, but operations continued until the operating theatre was hit.[24]

Leckrone and Robar were part of a shock team attached to Field Hospital No. 127, a unit of the Thirty-Second Division, when faced with artillery bombardment in July of 1918 at Château Thierry. Their role was triage, to stabilize those suffering from hypotension. "Despite every intention to keep hospitals and women out of harm's way," write Prior and Marble, "the circumstances of war and the practice of medicine brought nurses under the maelstrom of World War I artillery bombardments."[25] *The Stars and Stripes* magazine extolled how "nurses, smack up in the combat zone, will hold the 'frontest front' record for American women."[26]

BLOOD AND ANGUISH

The memoirs of those that held "the frontest front" share common topics and preoccupations from initial enthusiasm to baptisms of fire. Devastating wounds, unimaginable suffering, and immersion in work as an emotional shield mark out these testimonials. "Mademoiselle Miss" is quickly ushered into the experience of war near the front lines:

> But oh, I can't express what it means to hear the guns for the first time! It is a sensation so vast and lonely and crowded and cosmic all at once that one seems born into a new phase of existence where the old ways of feeling things do not answer any longer.[27]

Her 1916 book was written, then published, in order to elicit supplies and other financial support from those back home. Her "unique and inexpressible life" (29) is vividly portrayed in what is a relatively short text of one hundred pages. Not surprisingly for a book meant to encourage charity from America, numerous passages are devoted to illustrating the dire need for "platinum needles, big and little"(23), cotton and gauze, rubber gloves, ether, "dear little wash-cloths and hot water bags and rings, and oil-cloth and malted milk" (91): "I lack everything . . . cuvettes, glass jars, cups, oilcloth, syringes, needles, all in fact lacking but the pharmacy. *Ether is a memory here. Please* send the needles and all the other things" (28). She often describes nearly weeping at the sight of new parcels, "fresh blessings from our golden shores," and also "growing patriotic, to a degree I never knew in former days . . . a wee thrill that is quite peculiar, and makes me think that some day I may be a better American" (59). Van Vorst felt similar pride: "I think of America with an ever-increasing love; I am proud to belong to that young and far-off country."[28] While praising "all the generous donors," Mademoiselle Miss echoes Deland when she declares: "Why, daughters of France could not have done more!" (36). Although she notes that in her twelve-hour day she has little time for sleep and even less for "more than a hasty scrawl," she asserts that "actually for the first time in my life I begin to feel as a normal being should, in spite of the blood and anguish in which I move. I really am *useful*, that is all, and too busy to remember myself, past, present, or future" (18). Katherine Foote, whose 1919 memoir *Letters from Two Hospitals* was published under the pseudonym "An American VAD," experiences much the same, for although "it's such a great, terrible, sweet, sad world to live in, [it is] always wonderful, and I would not be doing anything else but this."[29] To be needed in and "useful" to a cause larger than oneself is a sustaining force in the midst of the "blood and anguish."

At times, however, particularly in the years before 1917, these useful and committed nurses express exasperation at their country's "fence-sitting":

> Wilson's last pipe-dream exasperates . . . me. Why doesn't he come over and see what he is talking about? He writes as if we were still dealing with the world as it was before the war. We are not—it's gone, over, and before the United States tries to make any further progress, that fact must be registered once for all. We find here a very appreciative, sympathetic and intelligent interest as regards the situation at home. They are tolerant and anxious to make every allowance for the difficulty of our position. It is felt, however, that Wilson must be under German influence . . . and there is even a canard that the present Mrs. Wilson is a Boche![30]

Foote's angry assessment of wavering US support is not atypical, though it is perhaps one of the more vociferous. Thus, when America does join the Allies in April 1917, she is ebullient. Seeing the Stars and Stripes hanging in Saint Paul's "fills her with joy that the great and glorious days of the new birth of our nation have come," and an article in the *Daily Telegraph* entitled "America at War" makes "proud reading nowadays." When "the band of the Royal Welsh Fusiliers struck up 'The Star-Spangled Banner,' there was tremendous applause, and you can't think what a feeling it gave me."[31] When at last "the papers here give one a splendid idea of what America is doing—her efforts and accomplishment" she hopes "everyone at home realizes what we are up against."[32]

As Foote asserts, no amount of reading or imagination, no amount of training, however professional, could have prepared America's daughters for what they would be up against: "One cannot describe it; one must see it to feel it. . . . Apart from the suffering, one's principal impression is that one has never seen so much mud caked on to human beings!"[33] Seeing a train empty itself of its wounded—grimy, disheveled, abject—at Amiens, Maud Mortimer similarly asserts: "Around this driftwood of war is certainly no trace of the glamour [of war]."[34] The enthusiasm Shirley Millard felt as her and her contemporaries' "hearts thumped to the tune of *Over There*," would be quickly dispelled. Yet:

> the lilt of *Tipperary*, *Madelon*, and *Roses of Picardy* heated my enthusiasm to fever pitch . . . I wanted to help save France from the marauding enemy. Banners streamed in my blood. Drums beat in my brain. Bugles sounded in my ears. I wanted to go overseas. . . . Knitting and selling Liberty Bonds [were] not enough for me. My imagination caught fire. I visualized myself driving an ambulance along the line of battle, aiding and comforting the wounded, or kneeling beside dying men in shell-torn No Man's Land. Or better still, gliding silently among hospital

> cots, placing a cool hand on fevered brows, lifting bound heads to moisten pain-parched lips with water. Reading to quiet men with bandaged eyes. Gently dressing a broken arm or leg. Or bearing the weight of a heroic convalescent as he took his first steps with a crutch.[35]

And, like other nurses including Vera Brittain before her, Millard imagined being able to nurse her boyfriend Ted, "oh, very slightly wounded . . . Gassed a bit, perhaps. Or with a sprained ankle. He would open his eyes and find me bending over him, my white veil brushing his cheek."[36] Such effervescent romantic ruminations starkly contrast with what she actually faces, her diary days later recording simply: "Terribly busy. It is all so different than I imagined. No time to write."[37] Looking back (her book combines diary transcripts with postwar recollection), Millard argued that "there was no need to write. The memory remains indelible."[38] The picture-postcard images of Florence Nightingales of the western front are unable to depict the gravity of the suffering. Thirty-five hundred hospitals are "filled with wounded." The quiet ward of imagination, where she fancies herself floating as a latter-day Lady with the Lamp, is replaced by:

> confusion, disorder and excitement . . . chaos. Nurses, doctors, orderlies, beds everywhere; yet not nearly enough to take care of the influx of wounded. . . . Hundreds upon hundreds of wounded poured in like a rushing torrent. No matter what we did, how hard we worked, it did not seem to be fast enough or hard enough. More came. It took me several days to steel my emotions against the stabbing cries of pain. The crowded, twisted bodies, the screams and groans, made me think of the old engravings in Dante's *Inferno*. More came, and still more.[39]

A cool hand on a fevered brow and the gentle dressing of a broken arm or leg are unwanted when "blood- and mud-soaked bandages" are removed to "find an arm hanging by a tendon." "Gashes from bayonets. Flesh torn by shrapnel. Faces half shot away. Eyes seared by gas" make a mockery of the tune that inexplicably "runs inanely through my head": "Roses are blooming in Picardy."[40]

Foote, too, describes "hideous shell wound[s] of the arm and hand," "dreadful" head wounds, stumps of legs, all of whose dressings "torture," resulting in "terrible agony." One man's wound, "after many fomentations and a fresh incision, has yielded up a piece of shrapnel about half an inch thick and a little less in length."[41] Mademoiselle Miss tells her family:

> I think you would sicken with fright if you could see the operations that a poor nurse is called upon to perform—the putting in of drains, the washing of wounds so huge and ghastly as to make one marvel at the endurance that is the man's, the digging about for bits of shrapnel.[42]

Maud Mortimer is even more unsparing in her depictions of the suffering she attempts to alleviate. Her memoir *A Green Tent in Flanders* (1917), with its deadpan, straightforward, unembellished prose, is very much like that of Enid Bagnold's *A Diary without Dates*. One man "has had a bad time with his knee. It seemed nothing at first but, after two operations, the articulation of the knee had to be opened. With forceps I hold the desolate flap while the pus is cleaned away and disinfectants poured on the wound."[43] Another has:

> [a] bad case of gas gangrene, and the doctors pass the fatal verdict: "*Faut te couper la jambe*." He refuses at first then consents; it is his only thread of chance. DePrecy amputates the leg at the hip joint, a staggering operation. The beauty of the mutilated body lying on the table and the severed leg carried away to be dissected is almost intolerable.[44]

And another young soldier has "a bullet through the spleen and kidney, half-flayed, with stomach, liver, and part of his intestines laid impudently bare, drains in the abdominal cavity and in his back."[45] In the chapter entitled "The Eye" we are told about Mongodin, the soldier of whom all you could see was his eye, which had a "brave smile":

> His wound was just above the left temple—a triangular-shaped hole almost an inch wide on its upper side. The projectile had passed behind the left eye . . . had opened way down behind the nose, and lodged rather forward in the roof of the mouth. It made his head seem like an empty hole. . . . The hour of his daily dressings was one for which I grew to time my visits to his ward. His nurse would allow me to pass her what she needed and, while the ordeal lasted, to engage the eye in conversation. The ordeal consisted partly in the excruciating change of *meches* and drains and in pouring through the gaping triangular temple wound streams of peroxide which would flow down behind the damaged left eye, behind the nose, and be caught by Mongodin himself, sitting up against his bed-rest, in a little white enamel kidney-dish which he would hold, without so much as wincing or even giving vent to any of those strange animal-like sounds for which the time being stood him instead of speech.[46]

We might apply Higonnet's assessment of La Motte's writing to that of Mortimer: "Unlike many wartime reminiscences that collect sentimentalized portraits of wounded soldiers these pages were not token bits abstracted for propagandistic or nostalgic purposes."[47] Such graphic description was no doubt part of an almost prurient attraction for readers of these memoirs and may have tacitly served the needs of propaganda for American involvement in this war against the barbaric Axis. But more importantly they reflect the author's need to release and to bear witness, "the peculiar predicament of the First World War nurses" that Santanu Das has identified. Das asserts, moreover, "If physical wounding and pain cannot possibly be shared, the

First World War nurses repeatedly dwell on acute body memories and body knowledge to establish a *physical continuum, a bodily bridge, as it were, over an ontological impossibility*: touch becomes the ground of both testimony and trauma."[48] Writing through the experiences to attempt to reconcile the double bind of being a healer but also an actor in a war generating so much suffering in the name of making the world "safe for democracy" was intrinsic to the American nurses' mental survival. Yet it was only a temporary solution. The suffering witnessed did take its toll. As Victoria Holder points out in relation to Alice Fitzgerald:

> She was beginning to lose all sense of compassion and feeling for her patients. They were becoming "stretcher cases, not human beings." To survive the atrocities, [she] had to lose her emotions and become numb to the despair. Only her training and dedication continued to push her forward. The physicians tried to excuse her from work, but she refused because she knew she was needed.[49]

In her published book, Fitzgerald notes when reflecting on the endurance of British Tommies to "stand the pain like super-human-beings," "it is best not to stop and think too much; one could never do the work."[50] Back in London, she was diagnosed with "a mild case of shell shock" and was close to a nervous breakdown. With rest, she recovered and was asked to train incoming British VADs at Boulogne. When the US entered the war, she requested to be reassigned to the American Red Cross. At the American Red Cross headquarters in Paris, she became friends with another American nurse, Julia Stimson. In her memoir *Finding Themselves* of 1918, Stimson is candid about her concern for herself and her nurses: "These frightful sights would work havoc with one's brain . . . what will we think when we get through with it all. How are we going to stand the mental strain?"[51] She admits, too, that "it isn't only the women that are affected by these things, the men [doctors] don't weep often, but they come near to it. And they get just as edgy." The understatement with which other nurses communicate their trauma is evident in Stimson's account, but the effect of the repetition of words such as *strain* reinforces the seriousness of the mental anguish:

> Our hospital is very full and we have many very bad cases. My nurses are beginning to show the effect of the emotional *strain*. Their nerves are a bit on edge, and I find that when they lose for a few days time-off-duty, as they all have been doing, they are not standing the *strain* and loss as well as they did the last time we were so busy. I have had about a dozen of them weeping. The continuous rainy damp weather, the accumulating emotional *strain* and the real hard work are having an effect on them that is bothering me. There is a convalescent hospital for Sisters at E. to which I can send one or two at a time for a short rest.[52]

Katherine Foote uses the same telling word: "Even with your big hearts and sympathy and imagination, you can hardly realize how terrible the strain is, nor how one longs for the end. . . . Only there's nothing for us all to do now but sit tight and work and fight until we win, even if it take all our lives; so uneasiness can have no lasting place in one's mind."[53] To "win" is paramount, and she admits that "if one did not have plenty of work to do, the contemplation of such suffering and the problems which the nations must deal with after the war would drive one mad."[54] Foote repeats the phrase "would drive one mad" in another passage when, after witnessing countless amputations, she exclaims: "Oh, the appalling, futile horror of it all! It has to be, but the longer one is in it, the more one is oppressed by the terrible waste of everything, from life downward, and to think of it constantly would drive one mad."[55] Such repetition reinforces the fear of succumbing to mental collapse. Work is the only antidote. Mademoiselle Miss, too, finds that relentless work sustains her:

> During the last week we have averaged 25 operations daily. One day we had 33, and if you have any conception of an operating-room where they are short of assistants, you may know the struggle, and the sense that one is saving bits from the wreckage, doesn't give one a chance to be mastered by the unutterable woe.[56]

She finds leave in Paris almost too much to bear: "I am ecstatic over getting back to work! Now that my Parisian fling is over, I might as well own that it was a terrific strain on my nerves. I discovered that a civilian life is unhealthy for me, and that I thrive under the banner of the Red Cross."[57] Rose Peabody Parsons asserts similarly that "it was slack times that were almost the hardest of all. When we were busy no one had time to think, and it was far better not to be able to wonder what it was all about."[58] It was necessary to protect the psyche, but Mortimer wonders, "Do I grow cynical of decorations? The price, these young lives, and the dear, boyish recklessness of their inexperience, are distorting my values." She comments, "How soon the priceless thin edge of deep emotion blunts."[59] Fitzgerald admits to similar desensitization: recognizing that she could often only treat the worst cases, she does so in a matter-of-fact statement that tells volumes. "The treatment was neither brutal nor indifferent. It was simply necessary."[60]

BEYOND THE ARMISTICE

When peace comes, Shirley Millard, though "glad it is over," finds "my heart is heavy as lead." Echoing Vera Brittain's reaction to the sounds of the guns in London heralding the Armistice, she recalls: "One of the girls came looking for me. They have opened the champagne for the staff in the dining hall. I told her to get out. Can't seem to pull myself together."[61] "Numb [and] bewildered" rather than joyous, Millard:

> felt a sudden shyness about returning home. I dreaded the curious eyes and eager questions. They would make a fuss. I knew that from the letters and clippings I had received. I shrank from the prospect of honors I neither wanted nor deserved. How could they know what *real* bravery, *real* heroism, was? I had seen it and wanted no chatter about it over teacups and cocktail glasses.[62]

Going home, though welcome for many nurses, was also traumatic and bewildering, far removed from the life they considered normal for so long, as Mortimer attests:

> A wire calls me home. Through a maze of conflicting emotions I look back along the days. Civilian life seems as far from me as a skin long ago sloughed off. After my breezy corner of a green shack, in this tiny world of keen living, how self-centered, and cluttered with artificial values that other life will seem.[63]

The psychological aftermath was to be revisited in the years after the war in countless ways. For some, like Millard, through publication, "a simple record of the dark caravan that winds endlessly through the memory of my youth."[64] For the majority, no doubt, silently. In a 1923 article for the *Atlantic Monthly*, Rose Peabody Parsons reflected:

> Memories of the war crop up. We suppress them. Books and articles dealing with the war we simply won't buy. We have had quite enough of unpleasantness. Yet we don't enjoy ourselves. . . . We think of those who bravely died. We think, too, of our dead selves who once vowed that these others should not have died in vain.[65]

Work again, was a necessary salve. Many women veterans campaigned for nursing reform and the promotion of their profession, like Fitzgerald. But surely most simply went back to "normal" life. Florence Hemphill returned to private nursing, settling in Kansas City,[66] although she wrote during the war that "I am certainly glad I came although I am afraid it will ruin me for ever doing private nursing again. It certainly isn't like anything I ever did before." Professional nurses felt that the lessons of the war should not be lost in peacetime: "let us pull together to save the best and finest things we have hoped and dreamed during the emotions produced by the great war, and let us carry over into an active and affirmative peace plans for the rescue and salvage of health, of morals and of a measure of human happiness."[67]

Julia Stimson went on to become superintendent of the Army Nurse Corps from 1919 until 1937. She was the dean of the Army School of Nursing for fourteen of the school's fifteen years of existence and president of the American Nurses' Association from 1938 to 1944. Her contribution to the multi-volume history of the US Army medical department documents the service of nurses from embarkation to demobilization, including those "found to be in need of rest or recuperation."[68] Such nurses were "sent to one of the rest houses for a reasonable period, or if in need of treatment, [were] assigned to one of the adjacent hospitals for the necessary care."[69] One hundred and thirty-four members of the Army Nurse Corps in the US died between 6 April 1917 and 11 November 1918, mainly from influenza or pneumonia, and were buried with military honors. In November 1918, a plot was designated for their internment in Arlington National Cemetery "if families so desired."[70] Four members of the Army Nurse Corps, attached to the first six units sent to France, died on active service; two were killed as a result of an accident on the SS *Mongolia*. None were killed by the enemy.[71] Stimson records:

> As was to be expected, although it is probable that such things were not in most people's calculations in connection with the war, a normal amount of accidents occurred among the nurses. One was killed in an airplane accident, another was run over by a train, another was thrown from a horse, and a number were killed in automobile accidents. Exercise of all sorts and diversions of every description were necessary and death under such circumstances was in the line of duty. It should be noted that the proportion of suicides among the nurses was abnormally low. Of the 10,066 nurse in the American Expeditionary Forces, but one of them committed suicide.[72]

Stimson's matter-of-fact reportage leaves us wondering about the "but one" nurse who committed suicide; studying the memoirs gives us clues as to a possible motive. The realization that "wartime medicine not only saved lives but probably cost lives" and "prolonged it," for instance, was the reason given by one American nurse who "sent back her Croix de Guerre ten years after the Armistice."[73]

CONCLUSION: THE FIRST WORLD WAR AND ITS AMERICAN LEGACY

The upbeat image of the American home front in the First World War as projected by the great majority of wartime (as opposed to postwar) fiction, newsreels, and the now-iconic recruitment posters is only one facet of what is a complex and contradictory society at war. The experiences of African American women, in particular, have only recently received attention. Over a thousand African American nurses who were registered with the Red Cross were rejected for service with the army, although some eventually were allowed to nurse wounded soldiers from the segregated black regiments when these returned stateside.[74] *Two Colored Women with the A.E.F.* (1920) was an early effort to chronicle not only the service of approximately 150,000 African American soldiers who served in France, but that of the sixteen African American women who were attached to the YMCA canteens.[75] But more scholarly work remains to be done.[76]

Writing in 1917, James M. Beck displayed an evangelical spirit in language not entirely unfamiliar in the early twenty-first century when he declared that:

> The response to the call for either registration or enlistment is not enough. It is essential that America should go into this war with a feeling of heroic joy in again battling for the noblest principles of liberty and justice. To arouse this spirit, so essential to the successful prosecution of any war, is not an easy task. Weighed down by our traditions of isolation and taught for the last two years and more by the chosen leader of the American people that they had not just relation to or concern in the objects and causes of the great world war, it is not unnatural that the great masses of the American people, while loyally submitting to the call for service, are still bewildered as to their just relations to the stupendous conflict. The very soul of America is to be tested.[77]

The women who witnessed and attempted to mitigate the suffering generated by the twentieth century's First World War found that the intended outcomes of "battling for the noblest principles of liberty and justice" were not always easily reconcilable with the loss of life or the physical as well as the psychological casualties. The sense of purpose, the "heroic joy," and feeling "as a normal being should," as Mademoiselle Miss put it, were predicated on experiences replete with horror, with "blood and anguish." The impact of international hostilities on jejune American confidence was continually negotiated by the nurses highlighted here and by countless others who left no written record. Although separated in time by nearly ten decades, reconsideration of such non-canonical, non-self-consciously modernist or literary texts is, I would argue, highly topical. For as historians assess the current wars in the Middle East, these works can help us to understand "why Americans tend to embark on so many crusades and why they so often manage to trip over their own ideals in the process."[78] Recent wartime nursing memoirs from America's latest efforts "to fulfill its global mission" will, no doubt, invite comparison with those by an earlier generation of women,[79] "shaken with that same vibration of the shock and hideousness of it all."[80]

NOTES

1. *President Wilson's Great Speeches and Other History Making Documents* (Chicago: Stanton and Van Vliet Co., 1919), 29.
2. For an analysis of debates surrounding the War on Terror and the wars in Iraq and Afghanistan, see L. E. Ambrosius, "Woodrow Wilson and George W. Bush: Historical Comparisons of Ends and Means in Their Foreign Policies," *Diplomatic History* 30, no. 3 (2006): 509–43.

3. Fiction served similar ends. Mary R. Ryder demonstrates how Edith Wharton's *The Marne* and Dorothy Canfield Fisher's *Home Fires in France* "promoted American virtues while chastising American shortcomings . . . [in] the last historical moment in which Americans believed themselves capable of saving the world." M. Ryder, "'Dear, Tender-Hearted, Uncomprehending America': Dorothy Canfield Fisher's and Edith Wharton's Fictional Responses to the First World War," in *The Literature of the Great War Reconsidered: Beyond Modern Memory*, ed. P.J. Quinn and S. Trout (Basingstoke: Palgrave, 2001), 144.
4. A review of the government's official propaganda organization, the Committee on Public Information, is provided by Krystina Benson in "Archival Analysis of the Committee on Public Information: The Relationship between Propaganda, Journalism and Popular Culture," *International Journal of Technology, Knowledge and Society*, 6, no. 4 (2010): 151–64.
5. G. Bateson, *Steps to an Ecology of Mind: Collected Essays in Anthropology, Psychiatry, Evolution and Epistemology* (Northvale, NJ: Jason Aronson, 1987), 206.
6. Ambrosius, "Woodrow Wilson," 509.
7. S. Cooperman, *World War I and the American Novel* (Baltimore, MD: Johns Hopkins University Press, 1967), 19–20, 42.
8. Higonnet, *Nurses at the Front: Writing the Wounds of War* (Northeastern University Press, 2001), xiii.
9. "Thank you for 'The Hill-Top on the Marne.' It is a good experience, spiritedly sketched, and I like the lady's pluck. It was diverting to read English again after so long" (*"Mademoiselle Miss": Letters from an American Girl Serving with the Rank of Lieutenant in a French Army Hospital at the Front* [Boston: W. A. Butterfield, 1916], 94).
10. G. Atherton, *Life in the War Zone* (New York: New York Times, 1916), 16.
11. *Report of the Committee on Alleged German Outrages Appointed by His Britannic Majesty's government and Presided over by the Right Hon. Viscount Bryce* (London: H. M. Stationery Office, 1915).
12. M. van Vorst, *War Letters of an American Woman* (New York: John Lane Co., 1916).
13. Ibid., 62.
14. Ibid., 99–100.
15. E. A. Kuhlman, *Petticoats and White Feathers: Gender Conformity, Race, the Progressive Peace Movement, and the Debate over War, 1895–1919* (Westport, CT: Praeger, 1997), 37, 79.
16. Address of the president to his fellow countrymen, 16 April 1917, *President Wilson's Great Speeches*, 37.
17. M. Deland, *Small Things* (New York: D. Appleton and Co., 1919), 28, 30.
18. Ibid., 8.
19. Holder, "From Hand-Maiden to Right Hand." World War I—The Mud and the Blood," *AORN Journal*, 80, No. 4, (October 2004): 652–665, 657.
20. Ibid.
21. H. Fraser, *Women and War Work* (New York: G. Arnold Shaw, 1917), 258.
22. Stimson, "The Army Nurse Corps," *The Medical Department of the United States Army in the World War*, vol. XIII (Washington, D.C.: US Government Printing Office, 1927), 287–351, 307, 309.
23. C. F. Thwing, *The American Colleges & Universities in the Great War, 1914–1919: A History* (New York: Macmillan, 1920), 146.
24. Quoted in R. M. Prior and W. S. Marble, "The Overlooked Heroines: Three Silver Star Nurses of World War I," *Military Medicine* 173, no. 5 (2008): 495.
25. It is likely that Rignel, Leckrone, and Robar never knew that they had been awarded the Citation Star. No Citation Stars were ever affixed to Rignel's or Leckrone's Victory Medals. Citations and documents were only "occasionally

mailed to the recipients." Moreover, these women were probably not "among the approximately 10,000 service members who requested to have their Citation Stars exchanged for Silver Stars" (Prior and Marble, "The Overlooked Heroines," 495).

26. *Stars and Stripes* 1, no. 19 (14 June 1918): 7.
27. *Mademoiselle Miss*, 12. Further references are included parenthetically in the text.
28. Van Vorst, *War Letters*, 89.
29. An American VAD [Katherine Foote], *Letters from Two Hospitals* (Boston: Atlantic Monthly Press, 1919), 28.
30. Ibid., 9.
31. Ibid., 62, 65, 68.
32. Ibid., 98.
33. Ibid.,1.
34. M. Mortimer, *A Green Tent in Flanders* (Garden City, NY: Doubleday, Page and Co., 1917), 320.
35. S. Millard, *I Saw Them Die: Diary and Recollections* (New York: Harcourt, Brace and Company, 1936), 3.
36. Ibid., 4.
37. Ibid., 10.
38. Ibid.
39. Ibid., 11–12.
40. Ibid., 14.
41. Foote, *Letters*, 80.
42. *Mademoiselle Miss*, 33.
43. Mortimer, *A Green Tent*, 142.
44. Ibid., 144–45.
45. Ibid., 149.
46. Ibid., 186–89.
47. Higonnet, *Nurses at the Front*, xvii.
48. S. Das, "'The Impotence of Sympathy': Touch and Trauma in the Memoirs of First World War Nurses," *Textual Practice* 19, no. 2 (2005): 244, 257.
49. Holder, "From Hand-Maiden to Right Hand," 659.
50. A. L. F. Fitzgerald, the Edith Cavell nurse from Massachusetts, *A Record of One Year's Personal Service with the British Expeditionary Force in France, Boulogne: The Somme, 1916–1917, with an Account of the Imprisonment, Trial and Death of Edith Cavell* (Boston: W. A. Butterfield, 1917), 5.
51. J. Stimson, *Finding Themselves: The Letters of an American Army Chief Nurse in a British Hospital in France* (New York: Macmillan, 1918). Higonnet points to "the dilemmas faced in frontline nursing, where self-control and technical efficiency conflict with emotional involvement and the threat of hysteria" (*Nurses at the Front*, xvii).
52. Stimson, *Finding Themselves*, 92; italics added.
53. Foote, *Letters*, 47.
54. Ibid., 7.
55. Ibid., 63.
56. *Mademoiselle Miss*, 21.
57. Ibid., 94.
58. R. Peabody Parsons, "Have We Kept the Faith?," *Atlantic Monthly* (August 1923): 670.
59. Mortimer, *A Green Tent*, 112, 127.
60. I. Noble, *Nurse around the World: Alice Fitzgerald* (New York: Messner, 1964), 68.
61. Millard, *I Saw Them Die*, 110.
62. Ibid., 111.

63. Mortimer, *A Green Tent*, 239.
64. Millard, *I Saw Them Die*, 115.
65. Parsons, "Have We Kept," 666, 672.
66. She shared a house with five of her siblings and her widowed mother. She retired in 1963 and died 16 April 1979.
67. "The Profession of Promoting Health," *Public Health Nurse* 11, no. 1 (January 1919): 10–12. Reprinted in S. Abrams, "Go Down to Suffering and Raise It Up," *Public Health Nursing* 28, no. 1 (2010): 103–4.
68. Stimson, "The Army Nurse Corps," 309.
69. Ibid., 310.
70. Ibid., 311. Stimson also notes injuries: "One nurse lost an eye having been struck by shrapnel during a German air raid, another received a shrapnel wound to the face in another raid, though did not have to be relieved from duty it was so slight; another was wounded in the leg during a raid near Amiens" (323).
71. Ibid., 351.
72. Ibid.
73. L. van Bergen, *Before My Helpless Sight: Suffering, Dying and Military Medicine on the Western Front, 1914–1918* (Farnham, VT: Ashgate, 2009), 356.
74. S. Zeiger, *In Uncle Sam's Service: Women Workers with the American Expeditionary Force, 1917–1919* (Ithaca, NY: Cornell University Press, 1999), 142.
75. A. W. Hunton and K. M. Johnson, *Two Colored Women with the American Expeditionary Forces* (Brooklyn, NY: Brooklyn Eagle Press, 1920).
76. Recent studies about African American soldiers include A. Lentz-Smith, *Freedom Struggles: African Americans and World War I* (Cambridge, MA: Harvard University Press, 2009).
77. J. M. Beck, *The War and Humanity: A Further Discussion of the Ethics of the World War and the Attitude and Duty of the United States* (New York: G. P. Putnam's Sons, 1917), xvii.
78. Cooperman, *World War I*, xiii.
79. "Appealing to the old American hope of 'freedom just around the corner,' both Wilson and Bush proclaimed American ideals to justify their new foreign policies. Whether in 1917 or 2001 or 2003, they led the nation into war, promising to protect traditional values and institutions at home and to expand these abroad, thereby making freedom and democracy the foundation for world peace. . . . They assigned a redemptive role to the United States, committing it to fight evil and create a new international order. After World War I, Wilson failed to make the world safe for democracy. His experience suggests that fighting wars to spread democracy and thereby attain perpetual peace is more likely to result in unanticipated costs and unintended consequences" (Ambrosius, "Woodrow Wilson," 542–43).
80. Parsons, "Have We Kept," 672.

Part II

Professional Identities

4 "All for the Boys"
The Nurse–Patient Relationship of Australian Army Nurses in the First World War

Kirsty Harris

The thousands of professional female nurses in the Australian Army Nursing Service (AANS) working overseas in the First World War experienced changes to many facets of their work as they nursed wounded and sick men often miles away from home. Australian authors Jan Bassett, through *Guns and Brooches*, and Rupert Goodman, through *Our War Nurses*, largely wrote Australian Army nursing "into being," providing a chronology of the progress of military nurses through Australia's involvement in overseas conflicts.[1] Their works highlighted the personal impact of war on nurses themselves against a background of military nursing administration and nurse movements.[2] Others have also written on Australian military nurses reducing the paucity of scholarly research into nursing and military nursing history in Australia, although publications are of an uneven quality.[3]

War transformed nursing practices and thus altered the relationship between nurses and patients. While the basic protocols for patient care learned in the nurses' civilian hospitals remained the foundation of their army nursing work, military organization and operation wrought change to almost every aspect of nursing. The clinical relationship changed as peacetime nurses learned to manage new types of war-wounds and unknown illnesses; consequently, so too did nurse–patient relationships. These relationships can be defined as having five recognized components—trust, respect, professional intimacy, empathy, and power. These components were often intertwined and variable. Drawing on diaries, personal narratives, letters, published accounts, and interviews, this chapter examines the changing nature of these components in the renegotiated relationships between Australian nurses and patients in the multination military environment.

WAR NURSING

From Australia's first major engagement in the war on 25 April 1915, nurses suddenly carried significant decision making in triage, first aid, and pain management. This significantly empowered Australian nurses and created the environment where male soldier patients had to increase their trust in the expertise of the nurse. Triage—the assessment, admission, classification, and distribution of military casualties for treatment—reversed the 'natural' order of care and overturned the nurses' ingrained protocol of helping the worst cases first. Now the least wounded and less sick received the earliest treatment, while those with the slimmest chance of survival were dealt with last. Many Australian nurses such as Margaret Edis learned and used the process of triage:

> What we were doing was standing there inspecting their wounds, if they were not soaked through, inspecting that they had had their anti-tetanus injection, if their condition was fit . . . If they were not considered fit they were drafted [to] the other side and their wounds inspected by the doctors or done.[4]

Although the number of nurses allocated to a military hospital was considered adequate, often the number was depleted or the bed number greatly increased, which made the situation unworkable.[5] The primary literature is littered with the nurses' dismay over staffing and the volume of wounded. Elsie Sheppard Cook's diary on 1 May 1915 noted: "we have got 700 badly wounded men and [only] six Sisters & Matron!"[6] Lack of time therefore limited the nurses' ability to properly treat the men let alone offer psychological and social support. Sudden large influxes of patients sorely tested nurses accustomed to the smooth working of a well-arranged hospital. Sheppard Cook also wrote: "simply running all day . . . & yet the awful feeling that they were not getting the right attention—simply impossible."[7] With such a workload, the nurses' balance of power over patients was reduced and communication decreased.

The vast majority of wounds—often multiple injuries—were caused by bullets, shrapnel, high explosive shells, trench mortars, and hand grenades. The meaning of the phrase *cannon fodder* was obvious to those nurses extracting pieces of shrapnel and bullets from mangled bodies. As in civil medicine, morphia was the most important pain management drug. Casualty Clearing Station nurses such as May Ashton often functioned with a high level of independence and used their discretion with pain medication and stimulant orders for their patients: "we give morphia & camphor, on standing orders, every 3 hrs if necessary without waiting for the MO [medical officer]."[8] This autonomy reflected the increased respect that both patients and other medical staff had for nurses.

The war empowered nurses in military hospitals in ways not previously conceived or expected. One way was in the saving of lives of many men weakened or injured by war through constant nursing work. One could call this work fighting nursing battles—as Sister Gertrude Moberly articulated succinctly: "14 officers for my ward, and some of them look like dying men, so we have some good fights with death ahead of us."[9] Sister

Beatrice Russell, alone on night duty during the German spring offensive of 1918, reflected:

> The Surgeons depended on us to let them know everything about the cases—I *know* that we really saved a lot of lives through noting that a case was going to bleed—was developing gas—and by tiding them over shock.[10]

Those nurses working close to the front line had to graduate from merely considering "methods of administering relief" to actually directing treatment, just as a doctor would do. In fact, military nurses were given the official right to "take such steps as may appear . . . necessary to meet the requirements of the case."[11] Nurse Kit McNaughton indirectly saved the life of a man from her hometown. Recognizing him in the mortuary ward (where patients were left to die), she intervened and had him removed to the operating theater for treatment; through her advocacy, he subsequently survived his wounds.[12]

A number of specializations developed during the war. Many Australian nurses served at No. 2 Australian Auxiliary Hospital in England, which became a special center for the fitting of artificial limbs for the thousands who suffered amputations.[13] An important part of this nursing role was helping patients cope physically and mentally with their missing limbs.[14] May Tilton reported that patients asked questions such as: "what is going to happen to me now, sister? What can I do with my life crippled like this?"[15] Offering reassuring answers increased the empathic relationship by nurturing faith and hope for a satisfactory postwar life.

Conversely, self-inflicted wounds were a confronting issue. Australian Army nurses in specialty British hospitals had to nurse self-inflicted cases who were prisoners awaiting court-martial.[16] Although considered a serious military crime,[17] it was hard to condemn the men without understanding the many conflicting influences. There is little evidence to show how Australian nurses responded, although it is likely that the nurses' trust and respect for these patients declined. Nurses learned to observe signs such as telltale powder marks to distinguish self-inflicted injuries, although occasionally they would confuse accidentally wounded patients with self-inflicted cases.[18] Some nurses saw it as part of their duty to hide the truth from the soldier's family by writing letters home that said the men had been wounded in action.[19]

Dealing with malingerers, who were consciously trying to avoid fighting by feigning illness, also reduced the nurses' empathy.[20] Malingerers often used the cover of a big stunt to get away in the rush and a massive shell dressing might only cover a mere scratch.[21] Ward nurses had to report any cases, and, after some experience, the nurses were usually able to distinguish the malingerer from the genuinely ill. Undeniably, military nurses thought poorly of those who wasted their precious time and resources.

Hope Weatherhead, nursing at No. 2 Australian General Hospital, found "the (lead swinger) the most trying and difficult to manage."[22]

PROFESSIONAL INTIMACY

In hospital, nurses became central figures in the soldiers' lives. Nurses reveled in their new role of being friend and personal confidante of their military patients. As historian Janice Gill highlights, the worth of army nurses must "be assessed in terms of their psychological value to the soldiers they nursed,"[23] and nursing in a war zone meant that the 'comfort' aspects of nursing grew in magnitude. Men generally admitted to base hospitals often had their stay measured in terms of weeks or months due to the combined effects of wounding and debility and the lack of quick-acting drug therapies.[24] Military nurses soothed, encouraged, and reassured their patients, waking them from nightmares where "they lived through all their awful experience again."[25]

Night duty became a new trial. Sister Anne Donnell discovered her patients feared sleeping and would seek her attention to put off 'lights out.' This created higher levels of intimacy:

> The boys asked for such little things to ease their pain—"This splint is loose. Could you bandage it up again please?"—"Sister, please give me some cotton wool to put under this strap."—"Have you got anything to put on this rash under my arms?"[26]

Florence James-Wallace, forced to leave her patients behind at the No. 61 Casualty Clearing Station in France when retreating in the German advance of March 1918, wrote of the noise they made in protest, and "it made us realize our being there meant more than the actual work we did."[27] Even during moments of great stress, such as a bombing attack on a hospital, wounded soldiers expressed their regard for the nurses. Sister May Tilton later wrote in her memoir that when she asked about the well-being of a patient with broken arms and a missing leg during a raid in France, he replied: "Sister, for God's sake, get under my bed! You might get hit."[28] In fact, military nurses often went beyond the call of duty both physically and emotionally to look after their patients.

Military nurses found ways to address the vulnerability and defenselessness that soldiers felt when hospitalized.[29] Historian Katie Holmes notes that depending on the patients' health, age, and nature of their wounds, nurses adopted different ways of relating to them.[30] The actual presence of female nurses was of inestimable psychological benefit and helped to allay patient fears of hospital.[31] Sister May Tilton, for example, boosted her patients' morale and validated and reassured them by praising "their courage, their grit and strength of will."[32] From the perspective of many soldiers, female nurses were proof that gentleness and compassion still existed in the war environment and they made more bearable the hideous realities of war.[33]

Military nurses thus tended to far more than men's physical wounds. Nurses' diaries and papers often include sentiments about their patients such as ministering to the soul as well as the body. They soothed and encouraged their patients, part of their work evolving into a mothering role.[34] Mothering was not difficult given that many soldiers were under the age of twenty-six; many were much younger. In addition, the absence of family in wartime strengthened the soldiers' need for their mothers' solace as Sister Jane Lempriere recalled:[35]

> As they come out of cholo. they all call for their ward sister like a lot of children calling for mother. The poor boys. I really don't know what they'd possibly do without the Sisters, we seem to be everything for the time.[36]

The female presence created a psychological link to home that male nursing orderlies or doctors could not as it was a gendered reaction by the soldiers. For many, nurses were the only female link with their homeland.

Operational requirements meant that the military sought to quickly discharge men from hospital and return them to the front, but for many nurses this was a point of contention. Sometimes they protected the soldiers, advocating for their patients' prolonged stay in hospital until they were physically and mentally strong enough to return to fight.[37] Some doctors applauded this advocacy: "How skilfully they work the unsuspecting [medical officer] and get their way—contriving that some tired, nervy boy shall get 'Blighty' instead of 'Convalescent Camp and the line.'"[38]

Nurses and their work represented change in the men's day-to-day routine as well as a link with their home lives. Grace Douglas noted the interest that soldiers took in the nurses doing everyday things: "Men, or boys as many of them were, were always dropping in to chat to us. They would watch us as we sewed or worked."[39] Military nurses deemed direct tactile contact—supportive touch—vitally important, as important as doing wound dressings, as it assisted their patients and eased their psychological pain. Soldiers, too, felt that a nurse's touch and soothing words took their minds "right off what was happening."[40] In direct contrast to rules in civilian hospitals forbidding nurses being familiar with male patients, the military nurses held hands, massaged heads, and kissed "their boys" farewell on their departure to other hospitals.[41] May Tilton noted how involved she felt in the task she performed:

> Saying good-bye to our patients was like parting from brothers. Some held my hand against their faces under cover of the bed-clothes, not uttering a word, while I stood silently, swallowing a big lump in my throat.[42]

As nursing historian Joanne Harding points out, the death of a military patient was different to a civilian patient because of the context in which it occurred and the role the military nurse played.[43] Sister Nellie Pike recalled these difficulties: "We could do little for some soldiers, except to help them die decently."[44] To die decently meant being pain-free and not alone.

POWER

Power was an issue confronting Australian military nurses daily, particularly in relation to military doctors and male orderlies and conforming to unfamiliar systems such as that of the British nursing services. Power in relation to military patients was affected by their military rank, the nurse's rank and perceived status, or the lack of it. As far as the military was concerned, nurses were officers and were not permitted to associate with lower-ranked soldiers. In September 1916, in an effort to control soldier–nurse relationships, orders came that the AANS had to wear military badges of rank, and Anne Donnell received a warning:

> Now that you Sisters have been given the rank of Officers and wear Stars you are not to go out with NCOs or Privates—or speak to them, excepting on duty. And if you do so you will be immediately sent away into a British Hospital.[45]

Many nurses had fathers, brothers, or friends enlisted in the ranks and felt that it was ridiculous that the army should prevent them from seeing the men purely because of differing status. Donnell reported that, in its short existence, the rule was "simply ignored by the majority," and an investigation showed headquarters had not issued the order.[46] This stance was crucial in helping the AANS create a relaxed environment for convalescent patients, particularly when they escorted the men while out of the hospital on picnics or tours.

Managing patients was a normal part of a ward nurse's duty. However, military status conferred new authority. As the patients' condition improved and they became convalescent, patients became restless with the monotonous life and it was hard to keep them in the hospital.[47] Soldiers with their already established camaraderie often conspired to thwart the nursing staff's disciplinary efforts. Some nurses had difficulty dealing with the propensity of convalescent soldiers to abuse their trust and absent themselves without leave.[48] However, like Australian military officers, they were also generally loath to report their patients' absences and misdemeanors.[49] Sister May Tilton resorted to the soldiers' honor to resolve her discipline issue and to rebalance the power between nurse and patient:

> I discovered, in one shack, three beds cleverly camouflaged . . . Before going off duty I unburdened my mind . . . I told them if they were

> not going to play the game I would be the one to suffer, for I would probably be sent away, as being incapable of managing my wards. The culprits immediately stepped forward and apologized, offering to go to the doctor and do the same. They did, and that was the end of the trouble.[50]

Nurses working with convalescents had to settle arguments between restless bored men suffering the long wait for transport home and make them obey the hospital rules.[51] Some had more success than others did in this power struggle. In the Convalescent Ward at 14 AGH in Port Said, Sister Nano Nagle apparently "had a way of her own of managing the boys and being their friend and nurse at the same time."[52]

TRUST

During the First World War, Australia provided only a small number of the medical units its army required overseas. Consequently, British medical services took responsibility for providing much of the medical aid for Australians. However, when Australian soldiers were sick or wounded, they had an intense desire to be in the company of Australian men and women and to be nursed and treated by them. Those the soldiers most trusted were other Australians, particularly the nurses, and with them they felt "like one large family," as Sister Effie Hargreaves remarked in a letter to her sister.[53] The nurses felt the same clannishness as the soldiers did, and this created a new form of patriotic relationship and a high degree of fellowship not experienced at home.[54]

A real and marked skill of the Australian nurses was dealing with the impact of the men's homesickness on their healing. Many nurses had brothers, cousins, and other relatives fighting and felt a close connection to them. To add to the trauma and stress of their work, from time to time a nurse would get word that a brother or close relative had been killed, badly injured, or made a prisoner of war.[55] Alice Kitchen declaimed in her diary on 5 May 1915 that the fact that Australian troops had gone into battle for the first time was a terrible strain on everyone. "There is so much personal element in it; if we had been nursing strange troops we may have felt it less, but among our own people the horrors of war are brought home to us more intensely."[56] Such a situation had the ability to unsettle and disempower nurses unless they had or developed the internal fortitude to stand the strain.

It is not possible to accurately determine how significant an effect on healing and recuperation the AANS had on sick Australian soldiers, but the number of comments in both soldiers' and nurses' diaries reflect its importance. Nurses used their knowledge of Australia and home to comfort, pacify, and amuse their Australian patients, particularly in British hospitals where the AIF were in the minority.[57] They sought mementos from home to bring Australia a bit closer for their Australian patients—gum tree leaves, pieces of yellow wattle, Australian newspapers, and comfort foods common in Australia. Individual nurses treated the soldiers as if they were their brothers, developing a relationship of mutual trust.[58] Jean Bisset, on a transport ship off the Dardanelles, was typical in looking out for AIF soldiers coming aboard. She reported one conversation in a letter home: "'I see you've got an Australian hat. Are you from Australia?' He showed teeth from ear to ear, and said, 'Yes, and I noticed your [rising sun] badge the minute I saw you.'"[59] Such meetings led to a great bond of sympathy, of affection, and of common duty between nurses and soldiers. The *Sydney Morning Herald* newspaper praised this close connection:

> To the nurse every mangled hero is a patient first. If a nurse's own brother lies beneath the surgeon's knife she may make no sign. She is there to do her work. On occasions she can use initiative where instant action is imperative to save life. Our boys love and honor her because she is one of themselves, doing her 'bit,' and understanding them so well. She knows their peculiarities, and enjoys their freedom of speech while admiring their patience and pluck under suffering.[60]

The Australian nurses helped to relieve loneliness from lack of family simply by being available to talk with their patients.[61] At Christmas, military nurses replaced relatives, playing Santa Claus and putting tins filled with sweets, handkerchiefs, and cards in each man's Christmas sock.[62] The nurses also organized birthday parties and concerts that the patients loved.[63] This solidarity and friendship created a high degree of trust that generally helped both soldiers and nurses to cope with the difficulties of their military life and countered the constant stress of observing death.[64]

One way in which military nurses garnered trust was by being a comfort to soldiers' families back in Australia, who suffered the uncertainty of not knowing what had happened to their loved one.[65] Many nurses, with their own family members on the battlefields, recognized how important information was to relatives, whether that was in Australia or in another country. Men trusted the nurses to write letters for them if they were illiterate or unable to hold a pen, and nurses read the replies to those patients who had lost their sight.[66] A ward sister always had letters to write in reply to concerned inquiries from anxious families. This new task often required creativity on the nurse's behalf, sometimes at the patient's behest, to minimize the severity of the patient's condition. May Tilton recorded that a very ill Scottish soldier asked her to write and tell his mother where he was, while being careful not to touch her fragile susceptibilities: "'Say I'm doing fine, and only got a bit of a scratch,' he said."[67]

EMPATHY

Part of the common understanding between nurse and patient developed through food. In many theaters of war, such as Salonika, Australian nurses ate the same rations as the troops, giving them excellent understanding of the frustrations and desires of the troops in regards to food.[68] Sister Nellie Pike was with No. 3 Australian General Hospital when it landed on Lemnos Island in support of the Gallipoli campaign in 1915:

> Army rations were crude, so were our cooks. . . . We kept ourselves alive by the Red Cross issue of Ideal Milk, tins of coffee *au lait*, Huntley and Palmer biscuits. We, in turn, kept our patients alive by the same means plus soup made from dried cubes and cooked over an open outdoor fire in a dixie, bully beef, army biscuits, salty bacon, badly cooked porridge, prunes, rice and straw. Straw was not an issue, it just got in during the cooking process. We had no bread, no butter, no margarine.[69]

Unlike most civilian patients, soldiers were malnourished and dehydrated when they arrived at hospital.[70] Rations, or the lack of appropriate variety, directly affected the condition of men and left them greatly susceptible to disease and debility.[71] It was certainly obvious to some nurses receiving patients, who thought the army "practically starved" the soldiers.[72] In hospital, providing invalid food for the men contributed to a new level of professional and social intimacy. While the question of food seems mundane as a nursing activity, Australian military nurses often struggled to feed their patients and even to find the right foods. Often the meal was not "invalid food" but whatever was available—and what the nurses themselves were eating. Sister Violet Hardwick lamented at Villers-Bretonneux that she could only feed the men "on hard biscuits, bully beef, and tea,"[73] wholly unsuitable food for sick men.[74] Such empathy for the stomach of the soldier patient was a defining difference between civilian and military nursing.

Nurses prepared and cooked their patients' teas, special diets for the very sick cases, and light diets all in their ward pantries, creating meals on their small and often recalcitrant primus stoves.[75] The nurses' resourceful attempts to purchase vegetables, fruit, and other items to improve the basic diet for their patients were adjudged outstanding. One medical officer was particularly impressed with the Australian nurses' generosity spending their own money "like water" to buy "goodies":

> How cunningly they contrive to get round food restrictions so that the boys shall have their due! "The boys have done their bit—the boys shall have their bit . . ." That's how they feel about the rationing of hospitals.[76]

Sometimes the nurses went direct to nearby fields and helped themselves. Sister Helen Chadwick, working on an ambulance train in France, sourced her patients' food from local crops and reported tongue in cheek: "We get our vegetables for the train when we can, as Fritz had planted acres of them for his own use."[77] Conversely, as Rachel Pratt had no green vegetables on Lemnos, she considered it appropriate to serve a bottle of stout to each soldier to aid their recovery.[78]

As matrons did not permit their nurses to visit stores or kitchens, nurses sought to provide their 'boys' with additional foodstuffs from outside the official system.[79] To make Christmas Day 1916 in France memorable for her patients, Sister Elsie Tranter recorded: "We are all becoming expert thieves and at every meal take what we can—sugar, nuts, etc., from the table for the boys."[80] Often this 'acquisition' aspect of their work, presented as 'surprises' for the men, generated much conviviality on the wards as well as aiding patient recovery, both physical and mental.

RESPECT

For most Australian nurses, the experience of nursing overseas during a war was an overwhelming psychological shock. The association with people of different cultures, races, and colors continuously combined to create confusion and changes over a very short period.[81] It is perhaps this area of service that most affected the nurses' levels of trust and respect for their patients. While they were prepared to serve the wounded of other nations, initially Australian nurses did not expect to spend long periods nursing non-Australians and they soon discovered that many were to work frequently in British hospitals and with other medical services.[82] Some were unhappy about the situation; others took a different stance, such as Sister Irene Bonnin, who wrote in her diary: "What does it matter who we nurse—we are all helping one another."[83] Generally, though, respect in a war environment appears to have been conditional on the nationality or color of the patient and was not openly given.

Some Australian nurses, meeting with new beliefs, values, and behaviors in stark contrast to their Western perspective, had their racist fears and prejudices strengthened in the Middle East. In Egypt, they nursed Serbians, and while working in Salonika, they learned much about the differing culture and behaviors of Greek, Italian, and Bulgarian patients.[84] Sister Gladys Walter in Salonika recorded: "One was surrounded by a confusion of strange tongues, weired [*sic*] customs and diverse stinks."[85] Her writing strongly reflected her perception that these people were not only inferior to her, but also dirty.

Some 450 Australian nurses found themselves replacing imperial nurses in British hospitals in India. They found this nursing unusual, challenging, and exciting but also frustrating.[86] The customs of Indian troops dictated "that by their religion their food must be prepared by their own people of the same caste."[87] Given that invalid food, both by mouth and per rectum, formed a significant part of medical treatment for diseases, this represented a large obstacle and altered the care that the nurses would normally give patients.

The language barrier associated with working in a non-English-speaking country with non-English-speaking hospital staff and patients was often a hindrance in providing basic care. In an effort to improve their communication with patients, many Australian nurses learned the basics of languages such as Arabic, Hindi, and French. If there was no common language, nurses had to rely on observation in the first instance, then sign language—no doubt a wealth of pantomime and gesticulation.[88] Nurses found the situation humorous at times and most overcame their difficulties by picking up sufficient words to make themselves understood.[89]

Nurses ran up against another set of cultural mores through nursing prisoners of war. In keeping with the nurses' professional code and the 1906 Geneva Convention, the Australian nurses nursed enemy patients.[90] Nursing the enemy wounded tested their highest ideals, especially near the front line in France, where nurses saw the state of their compatriots after their return from the trenches.[91] In many cases, nurses treated these prisoner-of-war patients with the same attitude, care, and kindness as Allied troops.[92] However, some nurses disliked the idea of looking after German prisoners, partly because of their own dislike of Germans and wartime allegations of German brutality, and partly because of prisoners' own attitudes.[93] Consequently, authorities often had to call for volunteers to nurse the thousands of injured or sick prisoners of war pouring into Allied hospitals.[94] Certainly, Australian Army nurses such as Elsie Steadman held a different attitude toward caring for prisoners of war, because she felt strange working in a barbed wire enclosure with guards, and equally because she felt morally authorized not to care about the enemy precisely because they were the enemy:

> Fritz made a good patient but I am sure he had not the fine sensibilities of our own British boys. . . . There was one thing about nursing them, you did your work without a vestige of sentiment, just for . . . work's sake, nothing else . . . Fritz you left when your day was done without a thought.[95]

To conclude, relationships between nurses in the AANS and their soldier patients during the First World War saw aspects of trust, respect, professional intimacy, empathy, and power between the two groups shift and evolve. Australian soldiers and Australian nurses created a 'family' relationship of trust and respect for one another in a strange and often chaotic environment, thereby helping each other to interpret and cope with the war. Professional intimacy increased with long patient stays in hospital, and the nurses' touch embodied a feminine presence in what was otherwise a male-dominated environment. A shared empathetic relationship between nurses and their patients was equally established through the food served to the men while in hospital, with nurses going out of their way to provide the best diet and variety that they could. The power balance between patient and nurse was affected by the introduction of rank to the nurses, while disciplinary action in the wards was dependent on the ability of the nurse to appeal to the soldier's 'best behavior.' While "all for the boys" was a maxim that most nurses worked toward, changes in clinical relationships, countries, cultures, language, food, and beliefs all played a role in effecting the renegotiation of the nurse–patient relationship. The nurses cared for patients of different nationalities and cultures, and they had to adjust both their nursing practice and their views in order to care for these patients, especially prisoners of war. The clinical relationship also changed when peacetime nurses had to learn to manage new types of war-wounds and unknown illnesses. Individuals' nursing practice was thus deeply marked in diverse ways by the experience of nursing overseas in 1914–1918. In the context of scholarly nursing history research, therefore, understanding the Australian military nurse–patient relationship adds a new and vital dimension to our understanding of military nursing during the First World War.

NOTES

1. S. Nelson, "A Fork in the Road: Nursing History versus History of Nursing?" *Nursing History Review* 10 (2002): 180.
2. J. Bassett, *Guns and Brooches—Australian Army Nursing from the Boer War to the Gulf War*, (Melbourne: Oxford University Press Australia, 1992); R. Goodman, *Our War Nurses: The History of the Royal Australian Army Nursing Corps, 1902–1988* (Brisbane: Boolarong Publications, 1988).
3. Other authors include R. Rae, *Scarlet Poppies: The Army Experience of Australian Nurses during World War One* (Burwood, NSW: College of Nursing, 2004); M. Barker, *Nightingales in the Mud: The Digger Sisters of the Great War 1914–1918* (Sydney: Allen and Unwin, 1989); P. Rees, *The Other Anzacs* (Sydney: Allen and Unwin, 2008).
4. Margaret Dorothy Edis, Interview, 25 July 1975, J. S. Battye Library of West Australian History, OH 96, 13.
5. A. G. Butler, *Official History of the Australian Army Medical Services 1914–1918*, vol. 3, *Special Problems and Services* (Canberra: Australian War Memorial, 1943), 555.
6. "Papers of Sister Elsie Sheppard Cook, AANS", Australian War Memorial (hereafter AWM), PR 82/135. See also Anne Bell, Diary, 1 May 1915, AWM41 1053; Sister Ella Jane Tucker, Diary, 29 August 1915, on board the hospital ship *Gascon*; Alice E. B. Kitchen, Diary, 30 April 1915, State Library of Victoria (hereafter SLV), MS 9627 MSB 478; Sister M. A. K. Wilson, Diary, 1 August 1915, AWM, PR 86/326; Sister O. Haynes, Letter, 24 July 1915, in *We Are Here, Too*, ed. M. Young (Adelaide: Australian Down Syndrome Association Incorporated, 1991), 62.
7. Cook, Diary, 2 May 1915.
8. Sister May Ashton, Letter, 18 August 1918, AWM, PR 88/25.

9. G. F. Hogan (née Moberly), *Experiences of a "Dinki Di" R.R.C. Nurse* (Sydney: Australasian Medical Publishing Company, 1933), 69.
10. "Report by Sister Beatrice Russell," 4. At No. 3 Australian General Hospital, March 1918, AWM41 1033.
11. "Standing Orders for Sisters," no date, AWM25 509/5, 2.
12. J. Butler, "Journey through War: The Great War Diaries of an Australian Army Nurse," (PhD thesis, La Trobe University, Melbourne, 2007), 269.
13. Miss Lily Gibson, Kellett Interview No. 33, AWM41 1072; Miss M. E. Cullen, Kellett Interview no. 12, AWM41 1072.
14. M. Tilton, *The Grey Battalion* (Sydney: Angus and Robertson, 1934 [1933]), 168; E. A. Eglinton, Letter, 13 May 1916, AWM, PR 86/068, 98.
15. Tilton, *Grey Battalion*, 83.
16. J. Butler, "'Very Busy in Bosches Alley': One Day of the Somme in Sister Kit McNaughton's Diary," *Health & History* 6, no. 2 (2004): 20, quoting "The War: General and Stationary Hospitals (from a Correspondent in Northern France)," *British Medical Journal* (22 January 1916): 141–42.
17. C. E. W. Bean, *The Official History of Australia in the War of 1914–1918* (Sydney: Angus and Robertson, 1941), 2:425.
18. B. Gammage, *The Broken Years: Australian Soldiers in the Great War* (Canberra: Penguin Books, 1975), 218, quoting Morgan, Diary, 17 June 1918; A. Thomson, *Anzac Memories: Living with the Legend* (Oxford: Oxford University Press, 1995), 39, quoting Alf Stabb, Interview, 7 September 1983, AWM, 12–16.
19. Gammage, *Broken Years*, 218, quotes Morgan, Diary, 17 June 1918, as saying that other medical staff also assisted soldiers to hide the signs.
20. Butler, *Official History*, 3:91.
21. R. Campbell Begg, *Surgery on Trestles* (Norwich: Jarrold and Sons, 1967), 123.
22. Sister H. Weatherhead, quoted in M. E. Clampett, *My Dear Mother* (Melbourne: Muriel Clampett, 1992), 154.
23. J. Gill, "The Origins of the Australian Army Nursing Service and Its Involvement in the First World War," *ANU Historical Journal* 15 (1981–1987): 67.
24. A. G. Butler, *Official History of the Australian Army Medical Services 1914–1918*, vol. 1, *Gallipoli, Palestine and New Guinea* (Canberra: Australian War Memorial, 1938 [1930]), 769.
25. B. Scates and R. Frances, *Women and the Great War* (Melbourne: Cambridge University Press, 1997), 22, quoting Tranter, Diary, 19 June 1917.
26. A. Donnell, *Letters of an Australian Army Sister* (Sydney: Angus and Robertson, 1920), 255.
27. Sister James-Wallace, quoted in Butler, *Official History*, 3:563.
28. Tilton, *Grey Battalion*, 253. At 47 British Casualty Clearing Station, Saint Sixte, Belgium, 27 September 1917.
29. Tilton, *Grey Battalion*, 206; M. Gurry, "Descent into the Other," *Age* (24 November 2001): 6.
30. K. Holmes, "Day Mothers and Night Sisters: World War I Nurses and Sexuality," in *Gender and War: Australians at War in the Twentieth Century*, ed. J. Damousi and M. Lake (Melbourne: Cambridge University Press, 1995), 46.
31. Holmes, "Day Mothers," 43.
32. Tilton, *Grey Battalion*, 114, 229.
33. E. H. Cuthbert, AWM41 958, 30; Gill, "The Origins of the Australian Army Nursing Service," 68.
34. Scates and Frances, *Women and the Great War*, 22, quoting Tranter, Diary, 19 June 1917; Miss Pringle in B. Abel-Smith, *A History of the Nursing*

Profession (London: William Heinemann Ltd, 1960), 5 quoting "Nurses and Doctors," *Edinburgh Medical Journal* (May 1880): 1049.

35. L. Robson, "The Origins and Character of the First AIF, 1914–1918: Some Statistical Evidence," *Historical Studies* 15, no. 61 (October 1973): 743. Robson states that 52 percent of his AIF sample were aged under twenty-five; K. Inglis, quoted in J. Lack, ed., *Anzac Remembered* (Melbourne: Department of History, University of Melbourne, 1998), 58; S. Austin and R. Austin, *The Body Snatchers: The History of the 3rd Australian Field Ambulance 1914–1918* (Rosebud, Victoria: Slouch Hat Publications, 1995), 4; J. Damousi, *The Labour of Loss: Mourning, Memory and Wartime Bereavement in Australia* (Melbourne: Cambridge University Press, 1999), 27; Hallett, *Containing Trauma*, 110, 198; Gill, "The origins of the Australian Army Nursing Service", 63.
36. J. Lempriere, Letter, 30 August1915, Alfred Hospital Nursing Archives, 6.
37. Tilton, *Grey Battalion*, 205; Goodman, *Our War Nurses*, 41.
38. "Our Sisters," *Una* (28 February 1919): 383.
39. Douglas, quoted in P. Adam-Smith, *Australian Women at War* (Melbourne: Thomas Nelson Australia, 1984), 27.
40. W. F. Adcott, *Genuine War Letters* (Melbourne: no publisher stated, 1920), 272. See also Tilton, *Grey Battalion*, 208.
41. P. Adam-Smith, *The Anzacs* (Melbourne: Thomas Nelson Australia, 1978), 334; Bassett, *Guns and Brooches*, 19.
42. Tilton, *Grey Battalion*, 185.
43. J. E. Harding, "The Role of the Australian Military Nurse during Operational Service," (PhD thesis, Flinders University, 2002), 10.
44. J. Laffin, *Damn the Dardanelles* (Sydney: Doubleday, 1980), 168.
45. Donnell, Letter, 23 September 1916, Mitchell Library (hereafter ML), MSS 022/1, 14.
46. Ibid., Letter, 20 January 1917; Tranter, Diary, AWM, DRL 4081A, 22. Tranter also recorded: "we don't take much notice of that rule."
47. Sister L. Smith, AWM41 1042, 1.
48. Sister A. Poole, "The Trivial Round," *Australasian Nurses Journal* 14, no. 11 (15 November 1916): 361; Donnell, *Letters of An Australian Army Sister*, 258.
49. Gammage, *Broken Years*, 255; J. W. Barrett and P. E. Deane, *The Australian Army Medical Corps in Egypt* (London: H. K. Lewis and Co., 1918), 62.
50. Tilton, *Grey Battalion*, 43; Gammage, *Broken Years*, 264–65, quoting Lieutenant R. C. Hunter, 2 Battalion, Letter, 8 April 1916.
51. Tilton, *Grey Battalion*, 105; Comber, AWM41 1072; E. Steadman, quoted in Bassett, *Guns and Brooches*, 68–69; Hardwick, AWM41 1072.
52. "Convalescent Ward Port Said," AWM27 373/61, 5.
53. Butler, *Official History*, 1:652; J. Robertson, *Anzac and Empire: The Tragedy and Glory of Gallipoli* (Melbourne: Hamlyn Australia, 1990), 203, quoting Private Willie Harris, 16 Battalion, Diary, July 1915, AWM, 3 DRL 7285; "A Touch of Nature Makes Nurse and Soldier Kin," *Herald*, reprinted in *Una* (29 December 1917): 316; Eglinton, Letter from No. 13 British Stationary Hospital, 29 June 1916, AWM, PR 86/068, 79; Edis, Interview, 13; Burns, AWM41 950, 2.
54. A. Donnell, Letter, 21 July 1915; P. Corkhill, Letter, 1 December 1916, quoted in E. Hain, ed., *Just a Few Letters* (Forster, NSW: no publisher stated, 1984), 14; Tranter, Diary, 14 April 1918; S. Macintyre, *The Oxford History of Australia, 1901–1942: The Succeeding Age* (Melbourne: Oxford University Press, 1986), 4:177.

55. An example is given in Cook, Diary, 12 April 1915.
56. Kitchen, Diary, 5 May 1915.
57. "A Touch of Nature," *Una* (29 December 1917): 316.
58. Staff Nurse Ada M. Willis, Letter, 1 August 1917, AWM, PR 01168/2, 116.
59. "Letter from Sister Bisset," *Una* (29 January 1916): 346.
60. "The Australian War-Nurse," *Sydney Morning Herald* (27 June 1917): 5.
61. "The War Diary of Sister Elsie Gibson," 28 January 1915; Lempriere, Letter, 30 August 1915, 2; Tilton, *Grey Battalion*, 68.
62. D. Armstrong, *The First Fifty Years: A History of Nursing at the Royal Prince Alfred Hospital, Sydney from 1882 to 1932* (Sydney: Royal Prince Alfred Hospital Graduate Nurses' Association, 1965), 109; Margaret Aitken, AWM41 937, 2; Donnell, Letter, 16 December 1915; Papers of Sister E. Davies, AANS AIF, Letter, 15 January 1916, AWM, 3 DRL 3398B, 3.
63. O. Haynes, Diary, quoted in Young, *We Are Here*, 45.
64. J. Lee, "A Nurse and a Soldier: Gender, Class and National Identity in the First World War Adventures of Grace McDougall and Flora Sandes," *Women's History Review* 15, no. 1 (March 2006): 94. Lee similarly relates how these relationships helped the British First Aid Nursing Yeomanry during the First World War.
65. Damousi, *Labour of Loss*, 17; S. Braga, *Anzac Doctor: The Life of Sir Neville Howse, Australia's First VC* (Alexandria, NSW: Hale and Iremonger, 2000), 178. See also Chapters 3 and 4 of P. Jalland, *Changing Ways of Death in Twentieth-Century Australia* (Sydney: University of New South Wales Press, 2006).
66. Young, *We Are Here*, 157; J. Durdin, *They Became Nurses: A History of Nursing in South Australia 1836–1980* (North Sydney, NSW: Allen and Unwin, 1991), 70; Holmes, "Day Mothers," 48.
67. Tilton, *Grey Battalion*, 184.
68. Laura Grubb, Letter, 8 July 1917, Oral Transcripts, Library and Information Service of Western Australia, A/11; Sister N. Pike, Interview, April 1950, quoted in Laffin, *Damn the Dardanelles*, 168.
69. N. Pike, quoted in J. Laffin, *Digger: The Legend of the Australian Soldier*, rev. ed. (Melbourne: Macmillan Australia, 1986), 64.
70. An AIF member in France, quoted in J. N. I. Dawes and L. L. Robson, *Citizen to Soldier—Australia before the Great War–Recollections of Members of the First A.I.F.*, (Melbourne: Melbourne University Press, 1977), 204.
71. See, for example, Gammage, *Broken Years*, 187, quoting Private T. J. Cleary, 17 Battalion, Diary, 1–3 November 1916.
72. Blodwen E. Williams, AWM41 1057; H. Weatherhead, quoted in Clampett, *My Dear Mother*, 147; Lempriere, Letter, 20 May 1915, 4.
73. Miss Violet M. Hardwick, Kellett Interview No. 39, AWM41 1072.
74. Butler, *Official History*, 1:249.
75. "First Major," "In Praise of the Primus," *The Kia Ora Coo-ee* (June 1918): 2; Sister Elfreda M. Doepke, AWM41 965, 4; Lieutenant Colonel J. W. Springthorpe, AIF, *Diary of the War 1914–1919: Medical Extracts*, Medical History Museum Collection, Brownless Biomedical Library, University of Melbourne, 69.
76. "Our Sisters," *Anzac Bulletin*, reprinted in *Una* (28 February 1919): 382.
77. Sister H. Chadwick, Narrative Account of No. 26 Amb. Train, AWM41 953, 2.
78. R. Pratt, "Nursing at Lemnos—August—December, 1915," *Reveille* 6, no. 12 (1 August 1933): 42.
79. Tilton, *Grey Battalion*, 55, 289; "Magnificent Story of the Australian Army Nurses," *Leader* (2 May 1931): 42; Eglinton, Letter, 8 October 1916, AWM,

PR 86/068, 86; E. M. McCarthy, Matron-in-Chief, British Expeditionary Force, Memo to Matron, No. 3 Australian General Hospital, 26 September 1917, AWM25 509/5.

80. Tranter, Diary, 23 December 1916.
81. This was the same for military nurses in many conflicts. See L. M. Van Devanter, "The Unknown Warriors: Implications of the Experiences of Women in Vietnam," cited in *Post-Traumatic Stress Disorder and the War Veteran Patient*, ed. W. E. Kelly (New York: Brunner/Mazel, 1985).
82. Bassett, *Guns and Brooches*, 66.
83. Durdin, *They Became Nurses*, 65, quoting I. Bonnin, Diary, 20 May 1916.
84. Butler, *Official History*, 3:572.
85. Goodman, *Our War Nurses*, 94, quoting Sister G. Walter, Diary, AWM; J. Beaumont, "The Anzac Legend," in *Australia's War 1914–18*, ed. J. Beaumont (St Leonards, NSW: Allen and Unwin, 1995), 172; Scates and Frances, *Women and the Great War*, 11.
86. Goodman, *Our War Nurses*, 81.
87. Sister G. M. Larkan, AWM41 995, 8; Sister Alma L. Bennett, AWM41 942, 8; E. Keast Burke, ed., *With Horse and Morse in Mesopotamia* (Sydney: A&NZ Wireless Signal Squadron History Committee, 1927), 130.
88. "Letters & Diary of Staff Nurse Laura Grubb", Staff Nurse Laura Grubb Letter to "My Dear Al" (232/89/18), no date, AWM, PR 83/40 (2).
89. "Experience of Miss E. M. Biggs," AWM41 943, 1.
90. Butler, *Official History*, 1:814; "The Sick and Wounded in War," *Hospital*, reprinted in *Una* (27 February 1915): 385.
91. Elsie L. Steadman, Papers, AWM, PR 86/302, 2; Cuthbert, AWM41 957.
92. E. C. Trestrail, "Three Months in France," *Australasian Nursing Journal* (15 June 1915): 190.
93. Gammage, *Broken Years*, 247; Dawes and Robson, *Citizen to Soldier*, 158–60.
94. Haynes, in Young, *We Are Here*, 26.
95. Steadman, AWM, PR 86/302, 2–3.

5 "Emotional Nursing"

Involvement, Engagement, and Detachment in the Writings of First World War Nurses and VADs

Christine E. Hallett

In both historical accounts and cultural representations of the First World War, there has been a focus on volunteer rather than trained nursing, particularly in Britain, where the Voluntary Aid Detachment (VAD) nurse has taken center stage. This imbalance owes its origins to a number of important influences. Firstly, VADs were much more likely than trained nurses to publish commercially successful accounts of their experiences. It was these accounts, rather than the more precise and pragmatic memoirs of trained nurses, that people wanted to read. The writings of individuals such as Vera Brittain, Irene Rathbone, and Enid Bagnold take classic romantic forms and offer their readers adventure stories and "page-turners."[1] Yet, the power of the VAD war narrative goes deeper than this. Her writings were well-received because the prevailing image of the VAD was an essentially positive one. The woman who nursed voluntarily rather than professionally captured the imagination of the reading public throughout the twentieth century. She was a romantic figure: her self-sacrifice, her willingness to forsake the comfort of the drawing room for the rigors of the military hospital, and her acceptance of the harshness of military discipline made her a classic mid-twentieth-century heroine. She was presented as an individual who knew the importance of her place in a rigid class- and gender-based society and was able to convey to her readers a sense of her nobility in stepping outside that place for the good of others. VAD-writers had much in common with middle-class combatant-writers such as Siegfried Sassoon, Robert Graves, and Edmund Blunden.[2] Their social capital, their class status, wealth, family connections, and educational opportunities enabled them to capture the market in wartime memoirs.[3] And so it was that they—not only because their works were readily available, but also because (albeit within the narrow confines of a particular class-consciousness) they were saying something about women's freedom to participate—were taken up by late twentieth-century historians and publishers and used to project a particular image of First World War nursing—an image that inevitably reflects only one part of the reality.

This chapter focuses, firstly, on the writings of three VADs and asks why they had such power for the generations that came after them. It examines one aspect of their experience: the way in which they viewed the emotional status and emotional role of the volunteer nurse in a military hospital ward. In order to do so, the chapter considers *Testament of Youth* (1933) by Vera Brittain, *We That Were Young* (1932) by Irene Rathbone, and *Diary without Dates* (1918) by Enid Bagnold. Clearly there were other influential works by VADs.[4] Yet, these three had a particularly strong influence on later generations. Their authors became household names for their association with wartime nursing. This chapter will consider how these three VAD-writers presented the emotional content of their nursing work in their texts. It will then turn to a consideration of the observations of trained nurses on this subject by drawing on professional writings, particularly textbooks and letters to the three professional nursing journals of the time: *British Journal of Nursing*, *Nursing Times* and *Nursing Mirror and Midwives Journal*.[5]

The chapter thus juxtaposes two very different types of sources, and this may be seen both as a strength and as a limitation of the work. The personal, reflective, and often partly fictionalized writings of the VADs offer us, in some ways, their deepest and most personal insights. Yet the impression of veracity is, inevitably, deceptive. Although they may be presented as exercises in "truth telling," these works may also reflect their authors' most highly fantasized imaginings. They were the productions of women who, in some cases, wanted to be viewed as romantic heroines, or who rewrote their war experiences according to the literary and ideological conventions of war memoirs set up by successful male combatant (or ex-combatant) authors, presenting themselves as an authentic "voice of experience" for their readers. The letters and textbooks of professional nurses—highly opinionated, yet practical and pragmatic in their style, always emphasizing "getting the job done well"—are an entirely different type of output: intended for a much smaller audience and presented as part of a problem-solving exercise. These professional nurses were writing for each other and were entering into debates about how they might overcome the professional and day-to-day working difficulties posed by the presence of large numbers of partially trained volunteers on their wards.

THE EMOTIONAL WORLD OF THE FIRST WORLD WAR VAD

Women such as Brittain, Bagnold, and Rathbone appear to have seen themselves as the soldier's friend and ally against the rigid regime of the hospital hierarchy—or at least they wanted to project themselves in this way in their autobiographical writings. They expressed a particular fondness for the "Tommy"—the common soldier. Irene Rathbone's *We That Were Young* contains a number of vignettes in which her heroine, Joan, falls foul of the senior nurses in her general hospital because of her kindness and leniency toward her Tommy patients.[6] A number of other episodes equally portray the VAD as kind and noble and yet politically naive and the hospital matron as the worst kind of unthinking bully, reinforcing outdated social etiquette and petty hierarchies. There also appears to be a generational clash, with the matrons in the VAD texts resembling the old men (both civilian and military) in the texts of male combatants: out of touch and indifferent to the younger generation's suffering. Take the following example:

> She was having a morning off, and was sitting on a bench beneath one of the plane trees in the hospital grounds writing letters. Lifting her eyes for a moment she saw Richardson hobbling along on his crutches in his blue hospital suit. (The "up" patients were encouraged to be out-of-doors as much as possible in this weather.) When he caught sight of Joan a broad grin spread over his face, and he paused as he came up to her. "Warm mornin', ain't it, Nurse?" he said. "My it don't 'alf take it out of you 'oppin' abart on these sticks!"
>
> "Better sit down a minute," she told him.
>
> He lowered himself on to the bench, and sat mopping his forehead, his bandaged foot sticking out in front of him. Joan, looking at it, wondered idly whether she couldn't, perhaps, in future, reduce the amount of dressing on it, so that it shouldn't look so ungainly, when a sharp voice calling "Nurse!" made her jerk up her head, and there, a few yards away, was Matron, walking rapidly from the huts in the direction of the main building. "Follow me, Nurse!" she commanded, without pausing in her course. And Joan, feeling rather weak at the knees, but without an idea of what was up, put down her writing-pad and followed her.
>
> Not once did Matron look round until she had reached her office, and then she turned on the girl and rent her. Under the stream of furious words with which she was deluged Joan gathered that she had committed an appalling offence in allowing a patient to sit beside her in the public grounds.[7]

This vignette, carefully composed to portray the VAD as a caring nurse and the matron as a ridiculous pseudo-military figure, demands to be treated with some care by historians and other analysts of discourse. The use of narrative tropes is so overt that it raises doubts about whether the author expected her piece to be viewed as serious historical documentation. She did, in fact, subtitle her book "A Novel by Irene Rathbone." Yet, there is evidence that she intended it to offer a "true" portrayal of the First World War VAD and her world. Lynn Knight has argued that while much of the writing is "hackneyed" and the dialogue "stagy," the books "merits a place in the canon of war literature." She further comments that it received critical acclaim in its day for its "realism and sincerity."[8] In her afterword to the same edition, Jane Marcus takes at face value the critique that presents the "military model" as the "undoing of the nursing profession" in which matrons belonging to a class below that of the VADs impose an unnecessarily strict discipline on them.[9] Marcus also, however, comments on the anesthetizing effect of the novel's sentimentality, which undermines the novel's apparent intention of portraying the suffering of a generation.

Far from sentimental, Enid Bagnold's autobiographical war memoir, *Diary without Dates*, is cool and detached in tone, mirroring the coolness and detachment of the professional nurses the author encountered at the Royal Herbert Hospital, Woolwich. This emotional distancing of the nurse from the patient's suffering forms a constant leitmotiv that runs through Bagnold's book, which is presented as a disjointed series of vignettes; each is written in a stark, repetitive, modernist style, intending to shock. As in Rathbone's, in Bagnold's writing the trained nurse is portrayed as harsh, unthinking, and judgmental:

> "I'd sooner be dead than lying here; I would, reely." You hear that often in the world. "I'd sooner be dead than—." But Mr. Wicks meant it; he would sooner be dead than lying there. And death is a horror, an end. Yet he says lying there is worse.
>
> "You see, I paid for a specialist myself, and he told me I should never be like this."
>
> There was nothing to be said . . . One must have one's tea. I went down the ward to the bunk, and we cut the pink iced cake left over from Christmas . . .
>
> I did not mean to forget him, but I forgot him. From birth to death we are alone . . .
>
> But one of the Sisters remembered him.
>
> "Mr. Wicks is still in the dumps," she remarked.
>
> "What is really the matter with him, Sister?"
>
> "Locomotor ataxy." And she added as she drank her tea, "It's his own fault."
>
> "Oh, hush, hush!" my heart cried soundlessly to her. "You can't judge the bitterness of this, nun, from your convent . . . !"[10]

Of all works that critique the detachment of nurses from their patients' emotions, Bagnold's is the most intense. The narrator's own curiously detached style seems to heighten the sense of the spiritual and emotional distance that exists between individuals in a military hospital. And perhaps here lies a clue to Bagnold's motive in writing the book. Her fascination with these issues highlights a deep-rooted fear that she herself will lose the capacity to engage with her patients' emotions:

> Pity is exhaustible. What a terrible discovery! If one ceases for one instant to pity Mr. Wicks he becomes an awful bore. Some days, when the sun is shining, I hear his grieving tenor voice all over the ward, his legendary tale of a wrong done him in his promotion. The men are kind

> to him and say "Old man," but Mr. Gray, who lies in the next bed to him, is drained of everything except resignation. I heard him say yesterday, "You told me that before . . ."[11]

Perhaps here lies the truth about the VAD's fascination with the apparent lack of emotion shown by trained nurses. It is rooted in the dilemma she herself faces between engaging meaningfully with her patients and risking becoming drained by their emotional needs. Lacking the training and experience of a professional nurse, the VAD is not sure how to handle this dilemma. Like Rathbone, Bagnold deploys realist techniques in her depiction of nursing, but hers is a harsh realism without any of Rathbone's sentimentalism. She inserts an apologetic preface into the frontispiece of her book: "I apologize to those whom I may hurt. Can I soothe them by pleading that one may only write what is true for oneself?"[12] Bagnold's own history is, of course, well-known. The publication of her book in 1918 led to her instant dismissal: her terse prose was *too* real, too immediate, and was viewed as a direct breach of confidentiality.[13]

The fears that find such oblique understated expression in *Diary without Dates* are openly discussed in Vera Brittain's highly acclaimed *Testament of Youth*:

> Although the first dressing at which I assisted—a gangrenous leg wound, slimy and green and scarlet, with the bone laid bare—turned me sick and faint for a moment that I afterwards remembered with humiliation, I minded what I described to Roland as "the general atmosphere of inhumanness" far more than the grotesque mutilations of bodies and limbs and faces. The sight of the "Bart's" Sisters, calm, balanced, efficient, moving up and down the wards self-protected by that bright immunity from pity which the highly trained nurse seems so often to possess, filled me with a deep fear of merging my own individuality in the impersonal routine of the organization.[14]

Brittain even suggests that trained nurses may have, in some sense, deliberately drained themselves of emotion. She comments: "There is something so starved and dry about hospital nurses—as if they had to force all the warmth out of themselves before they could be really good nurses."[15]

The motives for presenting oneself as the soldier's friend within the hospital setting are doubtlessly complex. Above all, VADs wished to present themselves as part of the war effort. They do appear to have had a need to be the comrades of their patients in a way that the trained nurses did not. Janet Watson has commented on the very different motivations of nurses and VADs, pointing out that the former took pride in their professionalism and the obvious achievements of their work, while for the latter it was participation in the war that motivated them.[16] It is for this reason that their identification with their patients could be quite intense.

At times, this camaraderie did shift, and VADs found themselves romantically involved with their patients. One attempt to convey a sense of the intensity of the romance that could develop between nurse and patient can be found in Irene Rathbone's description of the relationship between one of her characters, Pamela, and a handsome New Zealand officer-patient.[17] A more realistic (because based on a real attachment) and direct comment on the romantic feelings between nurse and patient can be found in Vera Brittain's reflections on how her work is driven by the fantasy that, in nursing her patients, she is somehow nursing her fiancé, Roland Leighton, by proxy—or indeed, that she may even nurse him in person one day:

> "I wonder," I wrote to Roland, "if some fine morning I shall come on duty and hear indirectly from a friendly VAD that a certain Lieutenant L. of the 7th Worcestershires came in with the convoy last night . . ." But it's too good to think of. It is the kind of thing that only happens in sensational novels.[18]

THE PROFESSIONAL WORLD OF THE TRAINED NURSE

Anne Summers has shown that the "militarization" of modern British society was a slow process that began decades before the outbreak of the First World War.[19] Among women, one of its most significant manifestations was large-scale volunteering for membership of VADs, which were established under the auspices of the British Red Cross Society and the Order of Saint John of Jerusalem in 1909. At the beginning of the war the VADs had about eighty thousand members and at its end about 120,000. Of these about twelve thousand were working as nurses in military hospitals and about sixty thousand in auxiliary hospitals.[20] Members of these detachments soon came—for the sake of convenience—to be referred to as "VADs." Among their most significant accomplishments were first aid, home nursing, hygiene, and invalid cookery, in which they could pass examinations and acquire certificates. Among their most highly valued traits were a higher level of educational attainment than most women of their generation and the ability to both improvise and show courage and "pluck."[21] These volunteers entered the world of the hospital—a world in which professional nurses had asserted their preeminence in the care of patients and the control of the environment. Carving out such a place had not been easy. The earliest professional nurses had frequently battled against the assumption that their role was merely to execute the regimes laid down by hospital governors and to follow doctors' orders.[22] Since 1887 they had been engaged in a battle for political recognition and a state register.[23] Although their status was clear it was by no means secure, and the presence of VADs in their domain of practice caused them much anxiety.

Unfortunately, some VADs appear to have shown a degree of insensitivity toward their professional colleagues, assuming that high social status conferred a natural talent that permitted them to overleap the intensive three-year training their professional colleagues had undergone and practice with expertise after a few months' experience.[24]

Even before the outbreak of war, complaints were appearing in the nursing press about the "invasion" of hospital wards by VADs. Take the following example from the *British Journal of Nursing*:

> To the Editor of the British Journal of Nursing. Dear Madam—will you allow me to ask through the columns of your valuable Nursing paper, whether other nurses feel as I do about the ladies of the Red Cross Society coming into the wards for an hour or so during the day? I am a second year probationer, and while I scrub the bath &c, these ladies are taken round by Sister (who I'm sure does not like it), and taught bandaging and small dressings. I object. Am I unpatriotic and narrow? I don't mean to be. But is it fair that these women should get the cream of the work, while we, who intend to give our whole lives to the work of nursing the sick, should lose the experience so necessary?[25]

Ethel Bedford Fenwick, Editor of the *British Journal of Nursing* and prominent campaigner for both female suffrage and nurse registration, was a strong advocate of a rigorous three-year training program for nurses. She inserted the following comment at the end of the published letter, encouraging others to complain publicly about the presence of VADs on hospital wards:

> This letter opens up a very wide question, and one which may have far reaching results in still further decreasing the supply of young women available for thorough training. This is not just the first complaint we have received as to the justice of the system. Others may wish to express an opinion on the question. We hope they will do so.—ED[26]

A paper presented by Mabel St Clair Stobart,[27] and subsequently published in the *British Journal of Nursing* weeks before the outbreak of war, offers an uncannily accurate prediction of the chaotic state of the nursing services at the opening of the conflict:

> In direct ratio to the discouragement given by the British Red Cross Society to the trained nurse, is the encouragement offered to the inefficient amateur who, with practically no qualifications, is welcomed in VADs, and smothered with lightly-earned brooches and medals, and given altogether false notions of her own value in national emergency . . . although the [Saint John Ambulance Association and British Red Cross Society] are excellent for teaching women an elementary knowledge of first aid, suitable for use in the street,

> and the home, in time of peace, the training is totally insufficient for the more serious emergency of war, in which discipline and a wider training are all important.
>
> It is not suitable that women who are to be called upon to take a share in the important work of National Defence, should in time of peace be under the control of philanthropic drawing-room Associations, and in time of war be suddenly transferred to military authorities who would exact thoroughness and discipline. Discipline is not learnt in five minutes. The duplication of authority is crippling in time of peace; it would cause chaos in time of war.[28]

One of the anxieties expressed by professional nurses was the fear that VADs would be willing only to do the work that interested them, rather than take on the more mundane tasks required to ensure patient comfort and the smooth running of a hospital ward. In August 1914, Ethel Bedford Fenwick invited Dr. Knyvett Gordon to make some comments on nurses' roles in wartime:

> All women nowadays are wanting to know how they can look after the wounded, for whom they feel so much sympathy, and many nurses will be helping with classes for instruction in these matters. To them I would say, Do not concentrate too much on First Aid, ambulance work, and so on. The walking stick and triangular bandage business is all very well in times of peace, but what is to my mind of much more important now is a little knowledge about germs and disease and the dressing of wounds, not omitting such measures as invalid feeding and cookery, which go towards the assistance of the patient's own blood corpuscles. It is better to know how to move a helpless patient comfortably in bed than to put on a bandage prettily.[29]

An anonymous column in the *Nursing Mirror and Midwives Journal*, for 22 August 1914, stressed the difference between "war fever" and "war spirit," commenting that:

> War fever has its origin in the emotions and appeals to every passing feeling as it is swayed by popular opinion and the latest rumor. The war spirit is founded upon the bed-rock of national character; it appeals to the intellect and the deeper forces that move men to action; it is indomitable and calmly severe, enduring with a dreadful patience to the bitter end if need be.[30]

The war fever was, according to this author, displayed most commonly among women who experienced a "sudden desire to become nurses" and had resulted in "hundreds of totally unsuitable candidates clamoring for admission to the ranks."[31]

By the winter of 1914, it was becoming clear to professional nurses that working with VADs was posing them with serious dilemmas. In early December, an indignant member of the Army Nursing Reserve wrote to the editor of the *British Journal of Nursing*:

> My experience is that some of these [Red X] are very dear girls, who really mean well, who get up at all hours to be on duty at six in the morning, but it is the whole emotional atmosphere of the wards which is so bad for them. I know my "Tommy," he and I have fought together for dear life in many a military hospital—in South Africa, India and elsewhere. He is a first class fighting chap, and recognises discipline and military authority without a murmur. But he is not used to be *drivelled* over, and when I see a pretty young girl leaning over the boys stroking their hands and smoothing their by no means fevered brows, I just want to tell that girl to run away and wash the dishes—a much more wholesome occupation.[32]

The anonymous writer, who referred to herself only as "Army Nursing Reserve" went on to comment ironically on how significant had been the absence of volunteer nurses from general hospitals prior to the war: "For all the years I have been a nurse never has there been any suggestion of society girls sacrificing any time to attend our poor sick in workhouses, infirmaries or elsewhere, to whom they might have brought so much brightness and comfort from the outer world."[33]

So-called "emotional nursing" was a phenomenon first identified in the winter of 1914 in an editorial of the *British Journal of Nursing*, which was probably authored by Ethel Bedford Fenwick.[34] The piece raised a flurry of correspondence in subsequent issues, most of which was in agreement with its views on the dangers of emotional entanglement in the highly charged environment of the military hospital ward.[35] One letter-writer commented on the powerful influence of social class in securing much-desired experience of training in how to nurse the wounded:

> It seems so incredible that after all the grinding and training, presumably trained nursing is a mere flimsy freak of the imagination and that anyone who chooses to don a nurse's uniform, however ignorant, is accorded professional rank. Indeed, one may add supremacy, as social status, not knowledge, is in reality the criterion for supervision.[36]

Concerns about the tendency of VADs to claim a greater degree of knowledge and insight than they actually possessed were expressed most clearly in the realm of emotional and psychological care. There was clearly a mismatch in the perceptions and expectations of trained nurses and VADs (or at least of those who wrote about their experiences). Each of the three classic VAD accounts examined here takes as a central theme a sense of the spirited, positive, and supportive camaraderie that existed between VAD and patient. By contrast, they are also, at times, highly critical of what they see as an unhealthy detachment and distance between trained nurses and patients. VADs felt they had a right to critique the apparent lack of emotionalism of nurses; trained nurses felt they had a right—even a duty—to critique the excessive emotionalism of the VADs, which they saw as a potential obstacle to a patient's recovery.

An inability to control one's own emotions was believed by many nurses to inhibit one's capacity to effectively support the patient. M. N. Oxford, formerly a sister at Guy's Hospital, London, published a textbook "for the inexperienced" in 1914. In it, she advised volunteer nurses to learn how to control their reactions to the wounds and pain they would encounter:

> A woman who means to nurse, especially in war time, must possess courage. The sight of blood need not alarm you; a very little blood makes a very great mess, and if you will set yourself to *help*, instead of gazing helplessly at the mess, you will nor be troubled by faintness not sickness. There is a great deal too in determining not to be frightened. The sight of pain is worse to bear; avoid worrying the patient by unnecessary talking or demonstrative sympathy, but help him as you can by fresh applications, altering his position or his pillows, or by gentle rubbing, if that is any relief. He will appreciate deeds more than words.[37]

Nurses who protested against the involvement of VADs in nursing work were sometimes supported by members of the medical profession. Bedford-Fenwick, in her influential editorial on "emotional nursing," quoted an address by Sir James Crichton Brown to a meeting of the Kensington District Nursing Association, in which he deplored the "merely affectional and emotional nursing" that was practiced when "under the agitated feelings created by the war, giddy women step in where angels fear to tread."[38] Bedford-Fenwick was notably—and unusually—able, on this occasion, to set aside her normally highly feminist sensibilities in order to quote the words of the influential doctor, which at first sight appear highly derogatory toward women. It seems that she shared his view that although trained nurses could exhibit the wisdom to "know the dangers to which the soldiers wounded in the defense of the Empire are subjected, if they do not receive competent care," VADs were mere "giddy women."[39]

MILITARY NURSING AND EMOTIONAL BOUNDARIES

Trained nurses saw "romantic entanglement" as potentially dangerous and disruptive, though some did, of course, later themselves marry men who had been their patients.[40] They expressed in their letters the anxiety that some women entered hospital wards with the deliberate intention of finding a lover. They believed that what they saw as inappropriate behavior of this kind could detract from the nurse's capacity to care well and effectively for all her patients. There is little in the writings of the three VADs presented here that would have allayed their fears. Irene Rathbone's at times overwrought depictions of the romantic intensity experienced by her characters go some way toward confirming the need for the "Sisters" to maintain safe emotional boundaries within the hospital ward environment.[41] Enid Bagnold describes how a patient was deliberately moved to another hospital because he formed a romantic attachment to her.[42] And Vera Brittain's understandable and honestly described emotional collapses following the deaths firstly of her fiancé and then of his close friend, to whom she had determined to become married,[43] bear out the pragmatic stances of hospital matrons whose perspective was generally that there was a job to do and a need for reliable workers to do it.

But considerations of professionalism went further than this. As nurse leaders began to form a sense of their own identity as the guardians of a developing set of professional standards, they were recognizing that a profession required its own clear code of conduct and its own sense of what would constitute "professional misconduct," although it was to be over seventy years before the profession's regulatory body would publish such a code and a further sixteen before personal relationships between nurses and vulnerable patients would be clearly prohibited.[44] Professional propriety was an overriding concern of nurse leaders in the early twentieth century and was probably all the more important at a time when the profession was nearing the end of its thirty-year struggle for a professional register.[45] The flooding of military hospitals with a semi-trained workforce was of serious concern because it undermined the arguments of those who had been fighting for a three-year training program and a single-portal entry to the proposed register.[46] Nursing—a mainly female profession, engaged in the highly taboo work of caring for the most intimate bodily needs of its patients—had much to prove.[47] In its not-too-distant past it had been a disreputable occupation suitable only for members of the servant class and tainted by association with women of "ill-repute."[48] Nurses were convinced that they had to work harder than members of other significant professions to demonstrate their standards of propriety and moral correctness.

Narratives of bullying in the memoirs of VADs have attained an almost mythic status. Yet it is unlikely that these bullying nurses formed more than a small minority of the profession. Both Vera Brittain and Irene Rathbone draw on their reminiscences of one particular matron: Rachael Cox-Davies, of the Royal Free Hospital, who, during the war, led the nursing services at the First London General Hospital in Camberwell as part of the Territorial Force Nursing Service (TFNS). Cox-Davies had had an interesting past as a military nurse on active service during the Second Boer War (1899–1902) and was to enjoy an illustrious future as an influential member of the soon-to-be-formed General Nursing Council.[49] She was clearly a remarkable and formidable woman. It is no coincidence that it was Cox-Davies who moved a resolution to the General Nursing Council in 1920 that "the Central Joint Committee [of the Red Cross and Order of Saint John of Jerusalem] be informed that VAD members who served in military hospitals are not eligible for registration."[50] After the resolution had been passed unanimously by the council, it was reported in the *Nursing Times* that the chairman had suggested a letter be sent stating "we very much regret that our answer must be in the negative." His suggestion was "met by a chorus of 'No regrets!'"[51]

The memoirs of Brittain and Rathbone suggest that Cox-Davies may, at times, have been harsh and controlling in her treatment of her staff (or, at any rate, of her volunteer staff). The historical record also, however, contains examples of caring and professional nurses who showed a marked camaraderie toward their volunteer colleagues. Dorothy Potts, VAD at the Second London General Hospital, Chelsea, wrote to her fiancé on 18 February 1917 of the "perfectly charming Sister" on her ward;[52] Miss K. Hodges, based on the Galician front, wrote in her diary that the English sister in charge of her ward was "wonderfully good and patient with my stupidity;"[53] and Margaret von Straubenzee, Red Cross VAD at Clandon Park Hospital, was sorry to leave at the end of the war, having enjoyed the encouragement she received from trained staff to develop her skills.[54] Similarly, Florence Egerton described in a letter to her mother the way in which the sister on her ward had referred to her as "simply a born nurse," and had urged her to enter nurse training.[55] Even *Testament of Youth* portrays a positive relationship between the experienced VAD and a professional nursing sister in a hospital in Etaples, Northern France.[56] Violetta Thurstan wrote in her *Textbook of War Nursing* of the need for trained nurses to exercise patience and endurance in their work with VADs. "What is most needed now," she remarked, "[are] fully trained nursing sisters . . . who can go on steadily day by day though most of the excitement and novelty has worn off, teaching batch after batch of raw probationers and orderlies, expending the very best of themselves on the various people with whom they come in contact every day."[57]

CONCLUSION: OVERLAPPING WORLDS

The writings of trained nurses, and particularly their letters to their professional journals, resonate with a sense of injustice and a feeling of insecurity. That untrained VADs, few of whom had shown any interest in nursing prior to the war, and many of whom were of significantly higher social standing than their trained supervisors, should walk into military hospital wards and assume responsibility for the most intricate and skilled of nursing duties was seen as an outrage by many. Quite apart from the fact that their demands for experience and practice denied valuable learning opportunities to probationers undergoing a full nurse training, there was a suspicion that these volunteers were more interested in obtaining a vicarious experience of the front line, in flirting with the wounded, or even in seeking a husband, than they were in contributing to the hard work of running a hospital ward or caring for injured and sick patients.

Various interpretations have been placed on the actions of both nurses and VADs. Some historians of nursing, such as Brian Abel-Smith, criticized what they saw as the shortsightedness of nurse leaders in their too-rigid closure of their professional boundaries.[58] When the newly formed General Nursing Council drew up rules for the admission of "bona fide" nurses to the new register in 1920, it took pains to ensure that those rules would exclude VADs. It is impossible to know how many genuinely enthusiastic and able nurses were lost to the profession.[59] Other commentators, such as Sharon Ouditt, have laid the blame for the tensions and hostilities between nurses and VADs more squarely in the hands of the latter. Ouditt observes that Katharine Furse, commandant-in-chief of the VAD, conducted a propaganda campaign to promote the worth of middle- and upper-class VADs at the expense of working- and lower-middle-class women, and that, in doing so, she unthinkingly denigrated those professional nurses who were obliged to work for a living and drove a wedge between two groups—trained nurses and VADs—who might otherwise have found some form of rapprochement.[60]

Many of these professional and class tensions were played out, particularly in the early months of the war, in the "emotional nursing" debate. Trained nurses valued emotional containment, believing that not only was such containment important for the well-being and healing of their patients; it was also what those patients desired. VADs, by contrast, perhaps because they found themselves so often cold-shouldered by trained nurses, felt that the whole environment of the military hospital was pervaded by coldness and detachment. They believed that they brought warmth, friendship, and camaraderie, crossing boundaries in the name of a unifying "war spirit," to this hostile environment.

There was, clearly, a mismatch between professional nurses' perceptions of VADs as romantic adventuresses and VADs' own self-perception as individuals who brought a spark of humanity to the harsh discipline of the military hospital ward. Nurses' tendency to critique what they saw as the frivolous behavior of the VADs was matched by the VADs' readiness to misinterpret trained senior nurses' attempts to protect patients from the dangers of emotional entanglement. A tendency to offer a negative critique of the perspectives and behaviors of the "other" pervades all of these writings. However, it remains vital to treat these perspectives critically and not to take at face value stories that may have been deliberately distorted for dramatic effect by authors who were, above everything, consummate storytellers.

NOTES

1. V. Brittain, *Testament of Youth* (London, Virago Press, 2004 [1933]); I. Rathbone, *We That Were Young* (New York, The Feminist Press, 1989 [1932]); E. Bagnold, *Diary without Dates* (London, Virago, 1978 [1918]).
2. S. Sassoon, *Complete Memoirs of George Sherston* (London: Faber and Faber, 1937); R. Graves, *Goodbye to All That* (London: Jonathan Cape, 1929); E. Blunden, *Undertones of War* (Chicago: University of Chicago Press, 2007 [1928]).
3. On social and cultural capital, see P. Bourdieu, *Distinction: A Social Critique of the Judgement of Taste* (London: Routledge, 1984).
4. See, for example, Millicent, Duchess of Sutherland, *Six Weeks at the War* (London: The Times, 1914); S. Macnaughtan, *A Woman's Diary of the War* (London: Thomas Nelson and Sons, 1915); O. Dent, *A VAD in France* (London: Grant Richards, 1917).
5. The *Nursing Record* was founded in 1888, was purchased by Ethel Bedford Fenwick in 1893, and was renamed the *British Journal of Nursing* in late 1902; the *Nursing Mirror* was also founded in 1888; and the *Nursing Times* in 1905. Full runs of all three journals are available at the Royal College of Nursing Archives, Edinburgh. The *Nursing Record* and the *British Journal of Nursing* are also available online from the Royal College of Nursing, UK. The *British Journal of Nursing*, edited by Ethel Bedford-Fenwick, prominent campaigner for nurse training and nurse registration, was much more likely to publish letters criticizing VADs than the other two journals. The *Nursing Times*, which had close associations with prominent members of the British Committee of the Red Cross, Sarah Swift and Sir Arthur Stanley, was the least likely to publish such critiques.
6. Rathbone, *We That Were Young*, 221–24, 229–31, 303–9.
7. Ibid., 222–23.
8. Ibid., xxi.
9. Ibid., 478.
10. Bagnold, *Diary without Dates*: 46.
11. Ibid., 60.
12. Ibid., frontispiece.
13. E. Bagnold, *Enid Bagnold's Autobiography*, introduction by B. Willard (London: Century Publishing, 1985 [1969]); Smith, *The Second Battlefield*, 72–77.
14. Brittain, *Testament of Youth*, 187.
15. Ibid., 211.
16. J. S. K. Watson, "Wars in the Wards: The Social Construction of Medical Work in First World War Britain," *Journal of British Studies* 41 (2002): 484–510; J. S. K. Watson, *Fighting Different Wars: Experience, Memory and the First World War in Britain* (Cambridge: Cambridge University Press, 2004).
17. Rathbone, *We That Were Young*, 160–69.
18. Brittain, *Testament of Youth*, 210.
19. Summers, *Angels and Citizens.*
20. Abel-Smith, *A History*, 85–86; Ouditt, *Fighting Forces*, 10–16.
21. For a contemporary account of the VAD movement, see Bowser, *The Story of British VAD Work.*
22. J. Moore, *A Zeal for Responsibility* (Athens: University of Georgia Press, 1988).
23. S. McGann, *The Battle of the Nurses. A Study of Eight Women Who Influenced the Development of Professional Nursing, 1880–1930* (London: Scutari Press, 1992).

24. On the tensions between nurses and VADs, see Watson, "Wars in the Wards"; Watson, *Fighting Different Wars.*
25. Anonymous, "Is It Just?" in "Letters to the Editor," *British Journal of Nursing* 53 (4 July 1914): 22.
26. Ibid.
27. Mabel St Clair Stobart was founder and head of the Women's Sick and Wounded Convoy Corps, the first British female unit to see active service during the First World War. Her views were staunchly feminist. See Smith, *The Second Battlefield*, 50.
28. Mrs. St Clair Stobart, "Women's Work in War," *British Journal of Nursing* 53 (18 July 1914): 53.
29. A. Knyvett Gordon, "Some Thoughts on the War," *British Journal of Nursing* 53 (22 August 1914): 156–57.
30. Anonymous, "The Nursing Outlook: War Fever and the War Spirit," *Nursing Mirror and Midwives Journal* 19 (22 August 1914): 397.
31. Ibid.
32. Anonymous, "Letters to the Editor," *British Journal of Nursing* 53 (19 December 1914): 497.
33. Ibid. This issue of 19 December 1914 contained a number of letters on the same theme, some of which expressed strong approval for a recent resolution passed at the Annual Meeting of the National Council of Trained Nurses protesting against "the danger of untrained nurses for the sick and wounded" (496–97).
34. Anonymous, "Editorial: Emotional Nursing," *British Journal of Nursing* 53 (19 December 1914): 357. It is likely that this editorial was authored by Ethel Bedford-Fenwick, although it should also be noted that many of the editorials in this journal were the work of the assistant editor, Margaret Breay.
35. One of the earliest editorials on the subject decried the tendency of the British Red Cross to send inadequately trained but socially influential ladies to serve as nurses close to the front lines in France, Belgium, and Serbia: Anonymous, "Editorial: Tinsel Glory," *British Journal of Nursing* 53 (14 November 1914): 377. The editor expressed clear approval for letters of protest against "untrained nurses" throughout the autumn and winter of 1914.
36. M. C. Patten, "Letter to the Editor," *British Journal of Nursing* 53 (19 December 1914): 496–97. See also: Sister Norton, "Everybody's Opinion," *Nursing Mirror and Midwives Journal* 19 (5 September 1914): 431; Anonymous, "Another Matron; Everybody's Opinion," *Nursing Mirror and Midwives Journal* 19 (26 September 1914): 481; Anonymous, "A Trained Nurse; Everybody's Opinion," *Nursing Mirror and Midwives Journal* 20 (10 October 1914): 29; Anonymous, "The Wrong Spirit; Nursing Notes," *Nursing Times* 12 (5 February 1916): 154; Anonymous, "A Wrong System of Training; Some of Our Readers' Views," *Nursing Times* 12 (12 February 1916): 177.
37. M. N. Oxford, *Nursing in War Time: Lessons for the Inexperienced* (London: Methuen and Co., 1914), 1–2. A similar tone is adopted by E. C. Barton, *Hints to VAD Members in Hospitals, Approved by the Joint War Committee of the British Red Cross Society and the St. John Ambulance Association* (London: Nursing Times, Macmillan and Co., 1915).
38. Anonymous, "Editorial: Emotional Nursing," 357.
39. Ibid.
40. Amy Stewart Hanssen was one such example. She married her former patient Osman Aldworth. His name appears in her autograph book, held by the Imperial War Museum. A. S. Aldworth, Autograph Album, Imperial War Museum, 03/43/1.

41. Rathbone, *We That Were Young*, passim.
42. Bagnold, *Diary without Dates.*
43. Brittain, *Testament of Youth.*
44. The United Kingdom Central Council's (UKCC's) "Code of Professional Conduct" was published in 1983: UKCC, *Code of Professional Conduct* (London: UKCC, 1983). In 1999 a further UKCC publication entitled *Practitioner Client Relationships and the Prevention of Abuse* stated unequivocally that "personal relationships with vulnerable clients are never acceptable": UKCC, *Practitioner Client Relationships and the Prevention of Abuse* (London: UKCC, 1999), 5.
45. Abel-Smith, *A History*; McGann, *The Battle of the Nurses*; A. M. Rafferty, *The Politics of Nursing Knowledge* (London: Routledge, 1996).
46. W. Hector, *Ethel Bedford Fenwick* (London: Royal College of Nursing, 1973).
47. E. Gamarnikow, "Nurse or Woman: Gender and Professionalism in Reformed Nursing 1860–1923," in *Anthropology and Nursing*, ed. P. Holden and J. Littlewood (London: Routledge, 1991): 110–29; C. Davies, *Gender and the Professional Predicament in Nursing* (Buckingham: Open University Press, 1995).
48. A. Bashford, *Purity and Pollution: Gender, Embodiment and Victorian Medicine* (Basingstoke: Macmillan, 1998); Summers, *Angels and Citizens.*
49. E. Bendall and E. Raybould, *A History of the General Nursing Council 1919–1969* (London: GNC, 1969).
50. Quoted by Bendall and Raybould, *A History*, 42.
51. Anonymous report, *Nursing Times* (2 October 1920). Cited by Bendall and Raybould, *A History*, 42.
52. D. Potts, 66 ms letters, Imperial War Museum, 3246 Con Shelf.
53. K. Hodges, Diary, 1974, Imperial War Museum, 92/22/1.
54. M. van Straubenzee, Diary, Red Cross Archives, LIB 88/595; T2 (STR).
55. F. Egerton, Papers, Red Cross Archives, 812/1–11.
56. Brittain, *Testament of Youth.*
57. V. Thurstan, *A Text Book of War Nursing* (London: G. P. Putnam's Sons, 1917), 13.
58. Abel-Smith, *A History.* On the introduction of VADs into general and military hospitals, see 85–88; on later shortages of nurses and the failure to recruit VADs to the profession, see 115–16; for a more general comment on what Abel-Smith sees as the rigidity of professional boundaries, see 241–43.
59. Bendall and Raybould, *A History.* On the rules for bona fide nurses and the way in which these affected VADs, see 41–43, 71.
60. Ouditt, *Fighting Forces.*

6 A Sister's War
The Diaries of Alice Slythe[1]

Janet S. K. Watson

Trained nurse Alice Slythe, of the Territorial Forces Nursing Service (TFNS), began two years' service in military hospitals in France in May 1915. From the start, she was very conscious of her diary as a record, as something for others to read, as something that documented something important—though she was not always sure just what that "something" was. Later, she gave the diary a title: "Sidelines of War." She also had an audience in mind; the diary was dedicated "to my sister Maud, for whom this diary was recorded." Though the dedication is in the past tense, suggesting it was likely a later addition, the language made it clear that Slythe was quite self-consciously addressing a reader, potentially multiple readers, rather than maintaining some form of internal conversation or personal reflection. It was intended as documentation of her war.

Slythe professed a clear conception of what her diary should be and made her expectations explicit from the first months.[2] In July 1915, she wrote:

> I'm being a little bit ashamed of this diary; far from being what you would expect of an Active Service Diary—it is simply an account, on the surface, of a pleasant summer holiday on the Continent; of course it *ought* to run "Called up at 2 a.m. dressed 50 cases; swallowed a cup of cold water; motored 3 miles up the lines; dressed 70 more; slept 10 minutes on a haystack" etc.[3]

The diary itself, however, rarely described the specific work she was doing, even when she was understaffed and overwhelmed. She could have produced the diary she theoretically described, when nursing at base hospitals and even more so when she was transferred to several Casualty Clearing Stations much closer to the front. That was not, however, the diary she wrote. Instead, she devoted many pages in multiple volumes to descriptions of her surroundings and her social life. She, like many others, was fascinated by the new technologies of war. She was drawn to the French countryside, first as picturesque and then as devastated. Slythe presented herself as a fearless adventurer in pursuit of physical closeness to the sights and sites of combat. As a professional, calm and capable, Slythe found her time in the wards less noteworthy than her excursions beyond their walls. She rarely described the work that occupied the majority of her time, and she was most likely to identify patients by their wounds, as cases and numbers and bodies rather than individual personalities; the exceptions to this tendency are notably fraught with emotion. Though at times distraught at being surrounding by deaths her professional expertise could not prevent, only once did Slythe question the war itself.

A few examples vividly illustrate the choices Slythe made to focus on the personal rather than the professional, the intimate rather than the epic. In late September 1915, after a gap in entries, she wrote, "And so I wrote no more for a fortnight!! Well, Princess Louise came round on the 18th & I had the joy of shaking hands with her: we have been pretty busy since then but I have managed two half-days with E." Those half-day adventures are then detailed at length when two weeks' nursing merited only the description "pretty busy."[4] Similarly, around three weeks later, Slythe wrote, "Nothing of much interest; we have been full up . . . & kept hard at it. However I have several fresh photographs so here they are."[5] The work itself, in many ways not fundamentally different from the work she had done in England (particularly while she was stationed at base hospitals), was not of enough "interest" for detailed description. Instead, the diary is jammed with photographs, some sketches, and many postcards, all documenting Slythe's new surroundings. The diary, therefore, is indeed not what she presented as "what you would expect," but it still proves to be a remarkable source. Rather than following some set model of what a war diary should be, it offers invaluable insight into the social politics and challenges of trained nurses working in military hospitals during the First World War. These women were claiming a certain professional status in the era just prior to the creation of the Nursing Register, which established guidelines and requirements for nurses, giving them official recognition as trained and skilled practitioners. They were also negotiating complex relationships among work, patients, medical staffs, and life. In the end, however, neither career nor the exigencies of war proved to be as important as conventional definitions of a woman's role, and Slythe left France and resigned from the TFNS to get married. Alice Slythe's evolving assessments of what was novel and what was routine, what was of interest and what was glossed over, what was paramount and what was not, complicate our visions of living through war.

BECOMING SISTER SLYTHE

Alice Slythe was born in 1883, the youngest of at least seven children born to Catherine Dunn over two marriages.[6] Catherine died when Alice was only ten, and it seems that her unmarried half sister and addressee for the diary, Maud Marsh, eighteen years her senior, took responsibility for her

(Slythe listed Marsh's residence as her home address during her war service). With no independent means of support, a career was a necessity, and Slythe probably trained at Croydon General Hospital. Mary Bird, principal matron, was on the Council of the TFNS, and Slythe followed Bird to the Second Eastern General Hospital in Brighton after the outbreak of war in 1914. An experienced professional who had just celebrated her thirty-second birthday when she began nursing in France in May 1915, Slythe was described by her matrons as "very satisfactory in every way" and "a particularly kind nurse, and an intelligent worker,"[7] and she was promoted to the rank of sister that autumn.[8] Slythe's status as a trained professional was very important to her; more than that, she believed that her quasi-military status as a member of the TFNS—or Terriers, as she often wrote—was a further badge of competence and skill. She delightedly recorded the comments of a former principal matron of the hospitals in the Boulogne area:

> It was she who told me that "the organisation of the T.F.N.S. is *sublime*. I get a batch of Sisters out; I look at them; & if they are Territorials I heave a sigh of relief. I know that their uniform is correct, their papers are in order, they have enough money, & *they know what to do*."[9]

This presumption of competence was key to the ways that Slythe portrayed her life in France. Hospital nursing was hospital nursing, and she was good at it; ironically, this meant that her diary could not be like the "active service" record she imagined. The work itself played a comparatively small role in her account, and the patients usually no significantly greater one. While Saint John's Ambulance and Red Cross VADs often described their work in painful detail, and sought out emotional individual connections with the soldiers in their care, Slythe's professionalism all but erased both wards and warriors from her account.[10] Though she presented her diary as an example of a known genre, what she wrote was in fact quite different, even when the material for the conventional war narrative was available to her. The nursing itself was still a known quantity, and Slythe's diary—like many—concentrated more on the novel than the familiar. What was new, of course, changed over the two years in France. Focusing particularly on the physical environment, her social life, her work, and the war, Slythe's two-year journey from base to Casualty Clearing Stations and back to base described an arc of strikingly changing perceptions alongside equally noteworthy continuities.

BASE

When Alice Slythe began her diary, she covered her pages with descriptions of what she saw, including romanticized views of France in wartime: "I'd like to take everybody I know in that tram, past the chateau & the lake with the picturesque boat house, through the sandy pine woods, past odd white cottages, past a big white house where the poilus are billeted." Quite typically, the page facing this entry contained images of the places she had been, in this case Hardelot postcards and a map clipped from a newspaper.[11] In those early days, the environment was a distraction from the work because France was more exciting than the hospital; as she wrote, "we started in to straighten things up but every ten minutes we were obliged to look out of the window as the outside world was so picturesque!"[12]

The first volume of Slythe's diary is crowded with images: photographs, rough drawings, diagrams, and especially picture postcards. She was eager to document her physical surroundings and wanted her readers to see where she was and what she saw. Slythe's landmarks were varied; on the same day she made note both of the "chateau taken by Lady Dudley (of the Australian Hospital)" and also that one could see "a little of the mud that Sister West fell into last night."[13] Slythe was also interested in churches and in religious practice more broadly. She commented regularly on the various services she attended, and she was delighted to be given the responsibility of fitting up the new mortuary with appropriate chapel-like accoutrements (some of which she sent to England for).[14] French churches, however—Catholic, presumably—were treated respectfully but as tourist sites, novel, exotic, not always in good taste. They, like beaches, woods, and chateaux, were the objects of sightseeing expeditions during off times throughout Slythe's time in France. When she had been there almost a year, she described an afternoon with a fellow nurse:

> We . . . came to a very small church which we explored. We found it wonderfully simple & dignified, no tawdriness anywhere & it looked more like the private chapel of a great house. Farther on we came to a perfect old grey house with a moat; how we should have loved to explore it. On the way back we got a basketful of cowslips, oxlaps, anemones & violets.[15]

The weather, the sights, the flowers—they were all the subjects of her outsider's eye of authority. Slythe "collected" churches as she collected flowers, but with longer-term expectations: she filled her diary with descriptions of their interiors and exteriors and wrote about the importance of finding just the right postcard views to include in her record of her war. Those postcards, however, were not the only items her shopping lists. One trip to Boulogne targeted not just "a p.c. of the Cathedral" but also "a bathing dress," a critical item for a socially minded nurse stationed near the beaches of Wimereux.[16]

There was, indeed, plenty to do and plenty of people with whom to do it. France had become almost a place of reunion for trained nurses; wherever Slythe went, she seemed to meet women she had known from training or hospitals in England, and they were her regular companions on half days and days off. "One is always meeting old acquaintances here," she wrote in July. And those encounters broadened the nursing network even further; she noted a month later that "I can't count how many mutual acquaintances I've discovered since coming out here."[17] The people mentioned most, in fact, are those with whom she worked. Some were merely referred to, but many of her coworkers—including the doctors and especially the orderlies—were described in detail. She told stories of the funny things they said, as when an airplane was described as doing "renaissance," and generally presented a bemused tolerance of their foibles.[18] These anecdotes were usually opportunities to demonstrate her own facility in French (and also German), of which she was clearly proud. They served, as well, as a means of establishing her educational superiority over the orderlies, who, as men drawn from the ranks, were unlikely to have had advanced schooling (or any medical training), but who, as members of the army, were not under the direct command of the trained nurses who ran the wards but were outside the official military hierarchy.[19]

It is clear that there was extensive social interaction among the men and women working in hospitals. "At Homes" hosted by both the nurses and the medical officers in turn were greatly detailed, down to the race Slythe won by carrying walnuts on a teaspoon across the room faster than anyone else—and the chic green Sevres china she won as a prize. When the nurses held a women-only costume party, their outfits were individually described:

> We are going to have a fancy-dress business tomorrow night—it will be great fun, as there is no time to get anything elaborate, so we shall just have to do what we can with what we've got. I see myself as a Chinaman with a fan & a pigtail, I have a specially favourite pair of blue pyjamas . . . We hear there are to be NO MEN admitted.[20]

Later she noted that apparently there had been an illicit male audience for at last some of the event, peeking through the cracks of the blackout shading on the windows.[21] More briefly, however, Slythe recorded that "Miss Ringland V.A.D. is engaged to Captain Bolt . . . this will be the fourth achievement in that line of 14 General since the start of war."[22] Though she was mildly critical of another nurse who seemed to have good friends among the medical officers wherever they went, Slythe, too, was ultimately engaged to a medical officer. Her conduct, however, was consistently described as "excellent."[23]

Wartime accounts written by volunteers in the hospitals displayed a number of consistent tendencies: the authors preferred nursing the wounded to nursing the ill, and they developed emotional connections to their patients. These volunteers, after all, had come to hospitals only because of the war; they had come specifically to nurse soldiers, to "do their bit." For professionals like Alice Slythe, however, the perspective was often different.

They were trained that high-quality care required efficient detachment, and while wartime nursing was exceptional, it was still, fundamentally, nursing; if there were no war, Slythe and her colleagues would still have been working in hospitals.[24] Slythe did not privilege soldiers as patients over other people who might be in need of her expertise, nor did she prefer the wounded to the ill. During her first year in France, she spent a significant amount of time nursing in the "Sick Sisters" ward—that is, nursing her colleagues from the area hospitals who themselves were in need of medical care. When her matron told Slythe about her impending change of duty, she was thrilled: "I am eventually to have Sick Sisters, which I shall love."[25] This was work she seems to have enjoyed but rarely described in detail.[26] It was not merely that she might have been reticent to discuss the illnesses of her compatriots—she at times showed herself entirely willing to do just that, as when she observed a surgery: "Sister had her operation at 9.30 a.m.; never saw such a crowd in the theatre: the Colonel was there; Col. Fullerton operated . . . Major Johnson assisted, also, Mr. Whittington . . . Mr. Venning & Mr. Coults, Capt. Brough anaesthetizing—& Sir Bertrand Dawson."[27] Discussing the medical issues was, however, also an opportunity for presenting what was new about it: Dawson was apparently "so keen on" the procedure "that he brought Ringland to *paint* the thing! Imagine it. In a *theatre* table covered with a sterile towel—paint brushes on it & a V.A.D. in a theatre gown to paint a gall bladder!!" That, for Slythe, made it "Active Service!"[28] In fact, she clearly preferred the Sick Sisters' ward.

Patients were mentioned most frequently in the diaries when they departed; they were described as leaving a gap in her daily life, but almost never as having filled any particular space while they were there. They were most often mentioned as an aggregate rather than as individuals; she recorded the numbers of patients arriving and departing far more often than she described any specific cases (and even then was likeliest to mention what was medically extraordinary rather than details of personality, circumstance, or background). Slythe was also explicit about the ways that patients were almost interchangeable; after one of the occasional lapses in her regular entries, she wrote: "Heavens, what a gap! & I don't seem to have been doing anything particular to fill up the time! Life has been quite peaceful; our floating population goes on as usual, people we have grown very fond of depart, & there's a gap, & then it gets filled up, & so it goes on."[29] "Gap" here referred both to people and to time, in almost equally impersonal ways. For an experienced hospital nurse, that essentially short-term nature of the relationship between the professional and the patient was expected. War or no war, occupants of hospital wards either healed or died; in either case, they did not stay.

Work, for Slythe, was in many ways what *least* merited discussion in her journals; she said so, repeatedly. When Slythe recorded in September 1915 the visit of Princess Louise and two half days out, she stated, "The rest of this fortnight has been just work."[30] That brief dismissal was not to imply that work was not difficult or important, but merely that it was not noteworthy. Slythe was a professional and took her job seriously, and it was often taxing. She was extraordinarily energetic; as she wrote, "I seem to do nothing but work [exceptionally hard] all the time I'm on duty & play tennis for dear life whenever I'm off."[31] If there was not enough real nursing to do, she could feel conflicted; soon after her arrival, she noted being "extremely pleased of course to know our Tommies aren't getting smashed; & one wouldn't have it otherwise, but scrubbing windowsills & methylating windows isn't quite the same work."[32] This gave her, however, more time to write; slow days made for long entries. In this case, Slythe's pen ranged through tennis, amusing evening promenades with the local population, sketches of the surroundings, descriptions of volunteer war workers, and the possibility of being moved to another hospital. She also explained the hierarchy among the different groups of women (Regular Army nurses, her own Territorials, the civil nursing reserve, and VADs). The politics of order and supervision could make all the difference for the work being done; as Slythe declared about the possible move, though she had heard the other hospital might not have a lovely location, "'they' also say that the Matron is charming, kind, & tactful; which is far more important to us than beautiful surroundings!"[33]

The relationship between the work and the war, however, was of necessity a troubled one. Slythe did not want soldiers to be wounded, yet how could she do her part for the war effort if they were not? Over the next several slack days, Slythe recorded "cleaning & turning out cupboards" and having "overhauled the stock of medicines & drugs."[34] However, as she wrote in a colleague's autograph album:

> But this is not the work that wins the praise
> Of cheering crowds down triumphal ways.
> And should the war end *now*, I shall not dare
> To show my face—just yet—en Angleterre![35]

Despite this verse, Slythe rarely directly connected her work and the war in her diaries. She did not focus on glory or honor, service or patriotism. Given the internal contradiction inherent in war nursing, there was a certain compartmentalizing that may have been necessary. She could write that "we are still waiting & watching for the Big Rush that, thank Heaven, never comes," but simultaneously be frustrated not to be doing the work she was trained to do and had come to France expecting to do.[36]

This mental segregation is also clear in Slythe's attitudes toward the technologies of war. As she wrote, "I hear from my sergeant that Zeps have been sighted making for England some time today; I hope they do no harm, but I would like just to *see* one!"[37] Their novelty pushed the machines of war into the realm of the tourist attraction, exciting rather than terrifying, at least from a distance. One evening, Slythe recorded "a beautiful yellow dirigible crawled over us about dinner time."[38] Playing tennis a couple of days later, she and her friends saw "the yellow airship [come] scouting round & an aeroplane above her! Unfortunately they were too far away or I would have taken a snapshot." That opportunity denied, she took a photograph of her friends instead, hoping to include it in the diary.[39] In the spring of 1916, they began seeing more airplanes; the shooting she repeatedly described as "being potted at," and the primary emotion she recorded was one of frustration that her coworkers were irritated when she pronounced "Taube" as a German word rather than Anglicizing it, as was the general practice.[40]

The most detailed description Slythe provided of a horror, in fact, was not really about the war at all. While she was in Wimereux, there was a fire in another hospital. Slythe called it "the most appalling thing happened, & I think it will haunt me for months," and devoted pages to it:

> There were clouds of smoke pouring out from three windows . . . we found nothing we could do except give the light of our torches to a few little groups who were looking after orderlies who had been knocked out by the smoke. Of course we were not allowed near the building.[41]

This fire was not the result of an air raid or directly related to the war; it was apparently caused by an electrical failure in a linens storage room that smoldered before bursting out and ultimately consuming the building. No lives were lost among patients or staff, but there were specific things that disturbed Slythe. First, it was clear to her that the British were better at fighting fires than the French, and so things were much worse than they should have been: "But the horrible part of the whole thing was the inadequacy of the fire appliances . . . As long as I live I shall never forget it—. . . that poor Tommy shrieking for water—& the accursed inadequacy of the French arrangements." The VADs billeted there lost their possessions, but the real loss, to a professional nurse like Slythe, was of the records, both those of the current patients and those from research done in the laboratory. Slythe's perspective on the fire was a combination of the analytical and the emotional: "Well, it's all over now, but none of us will ever forget it, & even now it comes back to me—& we can't pass that roofless horror without looking at it."[42] A traumatic event, to be sure, but—perhaps ironically—it was one that could have happened in peacetime as well.

This emotional distance should not imply, however, that Slythe was uninterested in the war. She and her colleagues certainly wanted to know what was happening, though rumors were easier to come by than confirmed news, despite official daily bulletins (one of which she pasted into her diary). Slythe also followed the war the same way that people home in England did: through the newspapers. Being in France did not give her access to appreciably more reliable information than she would have had if she had still been nursing in Brighton. She was, however, doing her job and seeing new things, and she was content to continue to do so where she was;

she articulated neither a desire for nor fear of being closer to the front lines. When, after more than a year of nursing in Wimereux, Slythe received new orders, she was initially dismayed. She and another nurse were being transferred to a CCS, as close to the front as women were allowed to serve. Slythe, however, did not represent this as a new opportunity to be more deeply involved with the war: "my orders came: the last thing on earth I expected . . . Matron was very sweet & said how extremely sorry she was. So was I."[43] She was disappointed to be leaving her well-established and comfortable situation, but not extraordinarily so.

CLOSER TO THE FRONT

Heading closer to the front, however, was not going to get in the way of seeing what there was to be seen, and Slythe listed in her diary the towns they passed through on the journey to the CCS. Along the way, Slythe and two fellow nurses missed a connecting train; they used the resulting delay to explore. This was not accidental: "I might as well confess that we missed the 8.50 on purpose, we argued that we might get gassed or anything & never see St. Omer at all!" They made sure to "explore the cathedral . . . which was very well worth it" (and was appropriately documented with postcards). Clearly danger still seemed distant, unreal; it was a convenient justification rather than something to be feared. Slythe was still in some ways a tourist of the war, excited to see "a Trench—only a reserve & unoccupied trench, but a trench nevertheless."[44] As she had a year earlier, Slythe was quick to establish her physical surroundings in her diary. The CCS operated out of a college in Bailleul (postcard attached): "We have the whole of the quadrangle with the exception of the church; the boys are still taught there." Slythe described the locations of the wards, including her own.[45] There were, however, some new constraints: fewer postcards were available (though she still found many and supplemented them with her own rough sketches), and she had less time to write. From the beginning, the work went at a faster pace and was far more intense. Slythe, the professional, was confident she could handle the situation, however: "I'd never dreamt of such work, much less seen it! But I managed to take hold all right, & really didn't feel very lost" when she took over her own acute ward.[46]

She was, however, even more interested the surrounding area than she had been in Wimereux. Now, her environs had the added interest of being part of the history of the war. "I cannot believe I am only a few miles from Ypres & Hooge & all those other places," she wrote, "so far I have only been to Locre," nearby—but across the Belgian frontier, so already something of an accomplishment. She had a tangible personal reason for feeling close to the sites of combat; a soldier she had nursed in Brighton had talked of the church at St Jans Capelle, and "I am only 2 ½ miles from St. Jans Capelle."[47] She was determined to mount as many expeditions to different locales as she could; as she wrote, "I mean to see just as much as I can of this country: if we are only up at a C.C.S. six months I am going to put as much as I can into it."[48] Battlefield tourism was not just a postwar phenomenon, but one that was practiced during the war itself.

Slythe began her explorations almost as soon as she arrived, with a certain disregard for military restrictions. Many of the entries were written at least a few days after the events they described; sometimes Slythe simply acknowledged the passage of time and the need to catch up, at others she backdated her accounts. In an entry dated 7 June 1916, she wrote, "I cannot catch up with this diary. There is so much to say & it is so difficult to remember it all."[49] Though Slythe described some social events comparable to those she had attended in the Boulogne area—the nurses and doctors held a "Book Tea," for example—more and more of her time off was spent venturing further into the surrounding countryside. By 10 June, she and another nurse had ventured into Belgium, heading down the Ypres road. Their first destination was the aerodrome, but then "we had a brilliant idea: to go on till somebody stopped us!" Slythe's attitude to regulations (and their violation) was somewhat uneven; she and her companion "decided not to publish our adventures, as we wish to see Locre again some day," but she also asserted that "next time I shall take my gas helmet; we are not supposed to move without them—& it was much on my conscience."[50]

She did not mention the gas helmets again, but she certainly continued her explorations. Only a few days later, "I was off [work] at five & started off by myself for Mont Noir," going by the interesting St Jans Capelle on the way. She was disappointed in her hopes of seeing Ypres from the summit, but still "had my first look at the Salient" despite being "misty & dull." Undeterred, she collected wildflowers for the hospital on her return. A tantalizing offer—"I met a field gun going up to Ypres, & the sergeant major said would I like to go too & I said yes I *would*"—led only to frustration when "they wouldn't take the responsibility," but it was still "a gorgeous tramp—& lots of adventures."[51] That sergeant-major may have been unwilling, but Slythe found other guides. One evening, she recorded:

> In a fit of sinfulness I decided to go to Neuve Eglise. Now the C.O. told me not to, as it was unhealthy. But when I reached the Ypres turning, for no reason whatever it struck me that Benediction at Locre might be rather nice. I hailed a lorry & fell on to it.

As she wrote defiantly, "who says I don't have adventures?"[52] Slythe continued to venture farther and farther during her off time, and became acquainted with some of the local military installations (and their friendlier officers).

When she was transferred to First/Second South Midland Field Ambulance in Warloy, she found even more opportunities. Her efforts culminated, perhaps, in early September 1916. Sisters Slythe and Brown went out together, determined to get closer to recent action, despite repeated attempts to dissuade them along the way. Believing they were hitching a ride in a passing ambulance, they ended up with a captain in the Royal Engineers on his way to make a daily report. Though the captain "tried to read us a lecture," Slythe wrote, "we smiled at him, & he took us up the road, & when he came to his H.Q. told the chauffeur to take us on to the top of the ridge & sit there for five minutes." On that ridge, they saw far more of the effects of the war than they had previously. There was nothing left of the villages of Ovillers, Contalmaison, La Boiselle, and Pozières except for a "collection of short irregularly spiked bits of wood sticking up 1–5 ft out of the apparently ploughed earth, & a few heaps of brick," or a "similar expanse of what looked like broken tooth comb." While they were still looking, Slythe wrote, "suddenly a huge cloud of earth sprang up into the air—My first shell-burst!" Among the horror of the sights there was still the excitement of how they related personally to her as a witness. The driver took them back down to the camp, where the captain, apparently no longer lecturing, continued their battlefield tour by taking them to Fricourt. There, they saw crowds of men, horses, and ammunition, and when they arrived in the town itself, "one low grey roof still holding together, & only 10 feet of that. Otherwise: for Fricourt see Ovillers." Their guide continued until "we saw a notice to the effect that persons proceeding farther—well—knew what to expect—so we turned back." The captain gave them some used cartridges as souvenirs and returned them to their door; they never even exchanged names.[53]

Slythe never again got so close, geographically, to the war being fought. Though she had found her way into Albert, she lost that access after, as she wrote, "some ass has come to Warloy with the tale of how two Sisters were at Albert yesterday, & a moment after they left, a shell came where they were standing & killed two horses & wounded three men; I wish people would keep their tongues to themselves."[54] The sisters had indeed been Slythe and Brown, and Slythe had looked forward to return visits, as "I am quite fond of Albert, & haven't nearly explored it enough yet." She was hoping the rumors she had heard that "the Huns have decided to reduce Albert to dust" were untrue; ultimately it was the British rather than the Germans who kept her away.[55] As she wrote later that month, "Haven't had any adventures."[56]

When Slythe wrote about her reported near-miss shelling in Albert, she expressed no sense of risk or danger averted, only irritation that the publicity would keep her from returning. There were only a few exceptions to her fearless self-presentation, dating from early in her time at Second CCS. She was very tangibly closer to the front lines, and while "bombardment in the day time, I don't seem to mind," she was having a hard time at night. Fitting her current experience into a more familiar category, she remembered a childhood book on the siege of Strasbourg during the Franco-Prussian War, and "once or twice lately I could fancy I had got into the tale myself!"[57] Working at a CCS was clearly an adjustment, and not just to the proximity of war in progress; Slythe found herself increasingly upset at work and writing about it in new ways. Her patients were dying, and, in too many cases, there was nothing she could do.

At first, she recorded the numbers: three dead in a day, fourteen in the first week.[58] Then came the first description of a death, that of a New Zealander; he arrived at the hospital already suffering from gangrene, and, despite the high amputation immediately performed, "he died out in the sunny garden at 1.30 p.m." This was "the worst thing since [the] war began" for her, and eclipsed the news about Kitchener's death that she recorded the same day. She still, however, could compare it to civilian life: "not since railway accidents at Croydon had I seen anything like it."[59] She continued to record the numbers of deaths, but also to do more.[60] On 16 June, after a quick social note and a comment about changing medical procedures, Slythe wrote, "Now I dive into horrors, so nobody who is squeamish need read any further." She then proceeded to describe, in brief but graphic detail, the extraordinary wounds of four men in her care. They were all alive, and she wrote nothing about them personally (other than one being "one of the prettiest boys I have ever seen"), but somehow she had to write about them. After those short paragraphs, she wrote, "But that's enough . . ." and ended the entry.[61]

It was not, however, enough. Later in the month she again recorded details of horrific wounds, and this time she added some personal details: the man who survived the bomb-throwing malfunction "is a dear big Irishman called Mulligan"; the boy with the serious skull fracture was Gates, "a little Cockney." Though she was writing about the living, it was death that was upsetting. "The other Sisters all say they are glad & thankful to see the men die when they are really desperate," Slythe wrote, "but I can not get used to it & I can't bear them all dying like flies, it seems as if we could prevent it & yet I know we can't." Again and again, her professional skills could not be enough. She had lost some of her carefully trained emotional detachment, and "even though" she knew that young Gates "if he lives . . . will never be normal, I don't want him to die."[62]

There was a tension within the diary entries; Slythe's emotional plea for Gates to live was immediately followed by a discussion (and postcard) of the organ in the local church and a lengthy account of "a jolly afternoon."[63] Similarly, another entry began with the large numbers of wounded and gassed soldiers treated both at her CCS and its Canadian counterpart and the "terrible number of deaths altogether." Slythe then went on at great length recounting a humorous visit to a former patient that had culminated in Sisters Slythe and Farmer spending "a strenuous time in the grass upon their faces, cajoling a guinea pig to come out from under a Company Office!"[64] And though Slythe accompanied another soldier to the cinema at the YMCA facility "to get right away from horrors," while there, she tried to convince a colonel to take her to Ypres.[65] Horribly wounded and (especially) dying men were "horrors"; the sites of the battles that had made them so, however, were not.

Slythe wrote several times about escaping during her time off work, but in varying ways. The day of her first view over the Ypres Salient, "as usual I set out to get miles away & happy again." She was not upset about the patients, however; rather, it was her fellow nurses who were bothering her, as "these women here occasionally rub me up the wrong way."[66] A few days later, though, she had another difficult day and described in detail the death of one of her patients. She then again started her next entry with "last night as usual I tried to get as far away as possible."[67] Her professional skills, faced with extreme situations, were tearing her in conflicting directions. She was proud of the work she was doing, though; after one particularly busy shift, with the floor so covered with stretchers that they could not move the supply trolleys through, she wrote that "it was the best morning work I've ever done," despite how frantic it had been (and how many had still died).[68]

Though professional pride stayed with her—she wrote later of one busy day with high numbers of soldiers coming through being "a very good piece of work"—the impersonal distance between nurse and patient continued to be broached.[69] Slythe still, almost despite herself, recorded horrific and personal details about the men dying while under her care and her frustration that she could not do more to save them. By the middle of the month, she was quoting letters from the mothers and sweethearts of the dead soldiers. Though there were fewer cases in the ward, the slower pace was a disadvantage, personally: "I think a rush would be preferable, as there wouldn't be time to think," she wrote.[70] Slythe seemed uncomfortable with her own new subjects; "well, that will do" signified her intent to change the subject, yet she continued. "It's the *helplessness* that hurts," she wrote, then described at length caring for a man likely to die but whose probable final hours had to be made more excruciating by denying him the water he craved because of the small chance he might yet live. Again, she tried to stop herself, this time successfully: "That's enough." She continued the entry by repeating a compliment she had received for her calm and professional behavior in the ward and by explaining that she hoped to get out and about again soon. Sometimes, perhaps, her "adventures" provided an escape from the wards, but recently she had not "felt like it"—"but if my people have a pretty good night to-night I shall go out tomorrow."[71]

This emotional battering led to Slythe's only antiwar statement. Up to this point, she had maintained a strict segregation between the suffering of the wounded and dying and the propagation of the war itself—so strict, as we have seen, that viewing battlefields could serve as an escape from the horrors of the wards. The closest she had come to criticism was at the beginning of July, when she "almost hope[d]" the rumored "huge attack" would not happen that night, "for it is our take-in day tomorrow & I do so *hate* to see them die."[72] At the end of that month, on another comparatively slow night that must have given her "time to think," Slythe wrote, "If the people who are responsible for the war could have a few nights on duty alone in this ward as it now is, they would stop it at any cost the next day."[73] This statement is striking in its distinctiveness; otherwise, Slythe focused almost entirely on her own localized perspective.

Slythe was moved from Second CCS on 9 August 1916, but she remained near the lines; she was sent initially to First/Second South Midland Field Ambulance at Warloy, and then, in October, to Eleventh CCS. The tenor of the diary, however, shifted significantly. Though she continued, as we have seen, to have "adventures," she regained her emotional detachment from the lives and deaths of her patients. She raised professional concerns, but not personal ones, about the soldiers. The field ambulance unit, she reported, saved 46 percent of their cases; she argued that they should be even closer to the line, as "it's the journey that does for most of them."[74] She had, perhaps, adjusted; she certainly returned to her fearless self-presentation. When the shelling came close to Eleventh CCS, Slythe mocked the idea of evacuating the nurses: "but I put on my wrist watch so that I should know what time it was if I *was* shelled!" She wrote that the "C.O. had thought we should be found all huddled together in the corner of one hut," when the nursing staff, seasoned professionals as they were, was taking the situation entirely in their stride.[75]

CONCLUSION: BECOMING MRS. ALMENT

On 25 November, after six months of nursing close to the lines of combat, Alice Slythe received orders for Second General Hospital at Le Havre. Slythe's return to nursing at a base hospital was anticlimactic for her diary, though not for her life, as it turned out. She nursed for a further six months before returning to England; near the end of that time, she became engaged to one of the medical officers, Captain Edward Alment, whom she married in 1917.

Slythe's time in Le Havre was very much like her time in Wimereux. She nursed in her hospital; she socialized with her friends and colleagues during her off time (and there was again a mostly hidden subtext of romance). She decorated the wards at Christmas time as she had the previous year. Shipping came and went in the harbor. The war continued. What had changed, of course, was Slythe's perspective. All these things were no longer novel and therefore no longer exciting. What had seemed so different, so worthy of pages and pages of documentation, now merited barely a mention; Slythe's entries became shorter, with longer gaps between them. In 1915, seeing France was compelling; for the six months from May to November 1916, she was compelled by seeing France devastated. A return to undamaged France, by contrast, seemed almost like a return to England. As Slythe wrote, explaining a two-week gap in entries, "There is really very little to write about here—the shipping in the harbour is the only interesting thing to look at."[76] She did not, however, write very much about even that, though she had found it worthy of repeated mention and several diagrams previously.

Entries became even more scarce in 1917; gaps grew from a couple of weeks to a couple of months. Though Slythe wrote that she had come "to the conclusion that it was my duty to continue the Diary if spasmodically only," the statement itself was a clear indication that the journal no longer served as an outlet for her views of her war.[77] Years later, thinking about possible publication, Slythe added a concluding comment to the diary: "I will end here. Life at one base is much the same as any other, so here I write FINIS." She cut into one of the last entries to make this ending, deleting a number of pages of additional postcards and descriptions. The very last entries are missing; Slythe later hypothesized that she had torn them out because they related to her romance.

Perhaps the most important thing that happened to Slythe in France—her romance and eventual engagement to Alment—is almost entirely absent from the diary. Though it was certainly novel, it was also, of course, intensely personal, which made it less appropriate for a document intended for the eyes of others (perhaps especially so in the case of Slythe's unmarried sister, Maud). Slythe immediately requested permission to resign from the TFNS, "my reason being that I am going to get married."[78] The war was far from over in May 1917; in fact, the summer battle season was getting under way. Demand for trained nurses was still high (especially ones who continued to have glowing reports), and Slythe was told by Sidney Browne, matron-in-chief of the TFNS, that "you can be granted two or three months' leave without pay and allowance if you would like to return to the Service after your marriage. If you decide to do this you can be posted permanently to a Home Station at the expiration of your leave." By contrast, Browne wrote: "if you resign you will forfeit your Gratuity and any other recognition of service which is granted to members who resign for reasons beyond their own control."[79] Slythe declined, however, writing "to request that I be permitted definitely to resign my appointment in the TFNS as I do not think it will be possible for me to return to the Service after my marriage."[80] Her request was granted, but reluctantly; Browne wrote that "the Advisory Council does not give permission to nurses to resign in War time but in the circumstances we will not stand in the way of your resignation."[81]

Alice Slythe chose marriage over war nursing, and in 1917, the TFNS clearly did not approve of what would in peacetime have been considered by many the proper role for a woman. After the war had been won, however, the TFNS and the War Office were less interested in condemning nurses for having made conventional choices and more concerned to laud the service of those whose accomplishments could enhance the reputation of the professionals. Slythe, now Mrs. Alment, was also happy to have recognition of her war work, and she applied for the "War Riband" to which she was entitled for her more than two years' service in France; two ribbons were sent to her in April 1920.[82] More than two years later, by then the mother of three, she was inquiring about the medals to go with the ribbons.[83] Bringing the story of her war service full circle, Alment was subsequently informed by Matron-in-Chief Maud McCarthy that "authority has now been obtained for the retention of the TFNS badge by those members who completed two years' approved war service." In 1917, Slythe had been required to return her badge as a consequence of her resignation upon marriage; in 1924, the badge was returned to her as "a memento of your war service."[84]

The stories of the war were changing, just as Slythe's diary had. The multiple endings left in the manuscript, retrospective, inserted and deleted, however, bring the diaries into focus as a palimpsest: simultaneous layers of what Alice Slythe thought she should write, what she did write, and what she wished she had written. Nurses and doctors, guns and planes, villages both picturesque and devastated, patients and wounds, all come in and out of focus in Slythe's record of her life. Those combinations are what render the diary so illuminating, bringing into focus the complexities and contradictions of a nursing sister's war. In the end, both the novelty and professionalism that were the primary themes of its pages paled in comparison to the more familiar story of love, domesticity, and the stability of marriage and family. During the war itself, those multiple narratives were in tension with each other, but only a few years later, they could comfortably coexist.

NOTES

1. I am very grateful to Mrs. Molly Currie, daughter of Alice Alment née Slythe, for permission to use her mother's diaries. I would also like to thank Christine Hallett and Alison Fell for their hard work and great patience as conference organizers and editors.
2. Much has been written about the conventions of both wartime and postwar narratives, including particularly the role of combat. See, for example, Fussell, *The Great War*; Winter, *Sites of Memory*; S. Hynes, *A War Imagined: The First World War and English Culture* (London: Bodley Head, 1990); and G. Mosse, *Fallen Soldiers: Reshaping the Memory of the World Wars* (Oxford: Oxford University Press, 1990). I have discussed many of these issues in Watson, *Fighting Different Wars.*
3. Slythe, Diary, 7 June 1915.
4. Ibid., 26 September 1915.
5. Ibid., 19 October 1915.
6. I am greatly indebted to Ann Fell for her genealogical research on Alice Slythe and her family.
7. M. Martin, 12 May 1915; L. Carter, 19 May 1916, TNA, WO 399/14532.
8. "I am walking round in new red stripes I only put on yesterday!" Slythe, Diary, 1 November 1915.
9. Ibid., 6 January 1916.
10. See A. Woollacott, "Sisters and Brothers in Arms," in *Gendering War Talk*, ed. M. Cooke and A. Woollacott (Princeton, NJ: Princeton University Press, 1993) 128–147; Watson, "Wars in the Wards." The classic account by a former VAD remains Brittain, *Testament of Youth.*

11. Slythe, Diary, 1 March 1916.
12. Ibid., 23 May 1915.
13. Ibid., 25 May 1915.
14. See, as examples, Slythe, Diary, 8 September 1915 and 2 January 2 1916.
15. Ibid., 1 April 1916.
16. Ibid., 7 June 1915.
17. Ibid., 14 July1915; 13 August 1915. See also 9 June 1915.
18. Ibid., 9 May 1916.
19. For more on the challenges of conflicting hierarchies of hospital ward and military structure, see L. Leneman, "Medical Women in the First World: Ranking Nowhere," *British Medical Journal* 307, no. 6919 (18–25 December 1993): 1592–94; Summers, *Angels and Citizens*. See also F. Murray, *Women as Army Surgeons: Being the History of the Women's Hospital Corps in Paris, Wimereux, and Endell Street, September 1914–October 1919* (London: Hodder and Stoughton, 1920).
20. Slythe, Diary, 13 June 1915.
21. Ibid., 15 June 1915.
22. Ibid., 13 March 1916.
23. Nurses were officially evaluated on conduct as well as on work responsibilities and capabilities. See Reports, 20 November 1915 and 30 May 1916, TNA, WO 399/14532.
24. I discuss these conflicting preferences and perceptions in depth in Watson, *Fighting Different Wars.*
25. Slythe, Diary, 13 August 1915.
26. Her matron reported that Slythe had "managed the sick sisters' wards very well indeed." TNA, WO 399/145532.
27. Slythe, Diary, 15 February 1916.
28. Ibid. Slythe's diaries are peppered with liberal use of exclamation points. When, much later, she considered publishing the diary, she crossed out most of them.
29. Ibid., 29 March1916.
30. Ibid., 26 September 1915; see also 1 August 1915.
31. Ibid., 12 September 1915; I have chosen not to reproduce her simile.
32. Ibid., 3 June 1915.
33. Ibid.
34. Ibid., 9 June 1915; 10 June 1915.
35. Ibid., 10 June 1915.
36. Ibid., 13 August 1915.
37. Ibid., 14 July 1915.
38. Ibid., 25 July 1915.
39. Ibid., 27 July 1915.
40. Ibid., 16 April 1915; 9 May 1915.
41. Ibid., 25 January 1916.
42. Ibid.
43. Ibid., 29 May 1916.
44. Ibid., 30 May 1916.
45. Ibid., 1 June 1916.
46. Ibid.
47. Ibid., 12 June 1916.
48. Ibid.
49. Ibid., 7 June 1916. At times it is difficult to tell the difference between a dated entry and a backdated entry. For the sake of consistency, I have used the dates Slythe recorded.
50. Ibid., 10 June 1916.

51. Ibid., 14 June 1916.
52. Ibid., 2 July 1916.
53. Ibid., 7 September 1916.
54. Ibid., 12 September 1916.
55. Ibid., 11 September 1916.
56. Ibid., 21 September 1916.
57. Ibid., 17 June 1916.
58. Ibid., 5 June 1916.
59. Ibid., 8 June 1916. A search of the *Times* validates her claim to have had experience dealing with rail and other accidents at Croydon. A particularly horrific rail crash in 1910, for example, resulted in seven dead and many injured, some needing amputations.
60. See, for example, Slythe, Diary, 13 June 1916.
61. Ellipsis in original; Ibid., 16 June 1916.
62. Ibid., 25 June 1916.
63. Ibid.
64. Ibid., 20 June 1916.
65. Ibid., 24 June 1916.
66. Ibid., 2 July 1916.
67. Ibid., 5 July 1916; 6 July 1916.
68. Ibid., 1 July 1916.
69. Ibid., 22 July 1916.
70. Ibid., 17 July 1916.
71. Ibid.
72. Ibid., 2 July 1916.
73. Ibid., 27 July 1916.
74. Ibid., 4 September 1916.
75. Ibid., 12 November 1916.
76. Ibid., 29 December 1916.
77. Ibid., 4 May 1917.
78. A. Slythe to M. Blakely, 30 May 1917, TNA, WO 399/14532.
79. S. Browne to A. Slythe, 20 June 1917, TNA, WO 399/14532.
80. A. Slythe, 25 June 1917, TNA, WO 399/14532.
81. S. Browne to A. Slythe, 3 July 1917, TNA, WO 399/14532.
82. A. Alment to War Office, TNA, WO 399/14532.
83. A. Alment (Slythe) to M. McCarthy, 17 December 1922, TNA, WO 399/14532. Christina Mary Alment (Mrs. Molly Currie) was born in 1919, Alice Margaret Alment in 1920, and Edward Anthony John Alment in 1922. Her son, known as Tony, was an obstetrician and gynecologist who was knighted in 1980 for his work as an advocate for women's health issues. His obituary in the *Times* mentioned that he was the son of a doctor, but, ironically, not that he was also the son of a nurse; *Times* (13 March 2002). By contrast, the *Guardian* mentioned both parents, but in a way that presented the war as a means toward romance rather than as evidence of her medical expertise, and it positioned Alice as Edward's wife rather than Tony's mother (28 March 2002).
84. M. McCarthy to A. Alment, 4 March 1924; A. Alment to M. McCarthy, 6 March 1924; M. Hogg to A. Alment, 2 April 1924; Reissued badge receipt, 4 April 1924, TNA, WO 399/14532.

Part III

Nurse as Witness

7 Negotiating Injury and Masculinity in First World War Nurses' Writing

Carol Acton

Eager to be sent to fight in France in early 1915, nineteen-year-old Roland Leighton writes to Vera Brittain of his frustration at remaining in England: "When men I once despised as effeminate are being sent back wounded from the front . . . can I think of this with anything but rage and shame?"[1] In April, soon after Leighton is sent to France, Brittain arranges to exchange her student status for the more culturally acceptable role for a young woman in wartime, a VAD nurse, suggesting to him "if you *must* get wounded, try & postpone it until August, by which time I might be efficient enough to help to look after you."[2] In October, nursing in London, she romanticizes to him the possibility of "Roland wounded & here! But it's too good to think of. It is the kind of thing that only happens in sensational novels."[3] This epistolary exchange reveals the extent to which the physical wound can become an abstract idea in the cultural consciousness: as capital in a country at war, the man can receive the wound, signifying masculinity tested at the front, while at the same time it creates his culturally acceptable counterpart in the woman who cannot be wounded but can participate in his wounding, and thus the cultural capital, by nursing him.

The wounded male body thus paradoxically reinforces gendered binaries and is a place where men's and women's war experience intersects. As Margaret Higonnet finds in accounts by Mary Borden and Ellen La Motte, their writing "joins the nurse and the soldier."[4] And Santanu Das claims of the physical act of nursing, "touching the wounds of soldiers is the most intimate way of body-witnessing history."[5] The wounded soldier's body and the nurse's intimate relationship with it thus provide a place in which we can examine these as interdependent narratives. Central to this interdependence is the particular burden carried by nurses wherein they must negotiate the fraught relationship between injury and the soldier's body in the context of complex and paradoxical constructions of wartime masculinity alongside the popular idealizations of the war nurse and of the soldier. This discussion thus focuses on how professionally trained and VAD nurses writing during the war and after confront and articulate this dilemma, as they find themselves caught between their need to bear witness to the injury the war inflicts and the equally urgent need to employ idealized wartime constructions of masculinity in an attempt to return dignity to the damaged soldier's body. Moreover, these women must also carry the burden of their own idealization in popular culture as ministering angels who, at the front, feel compelled to measure themselves against the stoic ideal they construct around their wounded patients.[6]

Leighton's equation of masculinity with a wound received at the front demonstrates his internalization of the relationship between the masculine ideal and the soldier hero, which Graham Dawson asserts "has proved to be one of the most durable and powerful forms of idealized masculinity," noting how "military virtues such as aggression, strength, courage and endurance have repeatedly been defined as the natural and inherent qualities of manhood."[7] If masculinity is defined in terms of physical strength and performance, then the wounded soldier is, as Trudi Tate asserts, "a paradox": "As a soldier he represented a powerful social ideal of manhood, yet the act of soldiering had damaged the bodily basis of masculinity, leaving him scarred, mutilated, paralyzed or blind."[8] The pressure exerted on men like Leighton, especially in the early months of the war, to accept and internalize mutilation as the price of masculinity was considerable, as Nicoletta Gullace affirms: "If the outward signs of the willingness to brave death—a uniform, a medal, a stump—had become the new symbols of masculinity, the potential mutilation of the male body was the price to be paid for the preservation of the masculine soul."[9] Joanna Bourke puts it even more directly: "The most important point to be made about the male body during the Great War is that it was *intended* to be mutilated."[10] For young men and women who had to face this "intention," accepting an ideology of masculinity that included mutilation might render the idea of it more palatable.

Unsurprisingly then, nurses' response to the wounded is conflicted. In contrast with Tate's representation of a damaged masculinity, women such as Vera Brittain and Irene Rathbone affirm masculinity through an erotic narrative that draws attention away from the damage of wounds to focus on the male body as an object of desire. Their postwar writings suggest that they draw on both the wartime ideal of masculinity as manifest in the wound and a postwar narrative of reconstruction in which the male body came to be idealized. In her discussion of the postwar male body, Ana Carden-Coyne points out that "physical rehabilitation [was] wedded to sexual virility."[11] As she argues, with the classically perfect male body integrated into war memorials, the postwar emphasis was on the relationship between war and the eroticizing of the male body, and especially the renewal of the wounded body. While Brittain could not have acknowledged it overtly at the time, writing her memoirs after the war she would admit the undeniably erotic, and thus for a nurse and woman transgressive, response that connects her potentially wounded lover to her intimate physical relationship with the wounded men in her care. A prewar culture that would not have given women permission to speak of male sexuality seems postwar to have allowed Brittain to acknowledge the erotic element in nursing and, perhaps, even to feel under a certain cultural obligation to claim it as a means of postwar restoration of virility to the wounded. Thus in *Testament of Youth* (1933) she writes:

> In the early days of the war the majority of soldier patients belonged to a first-rate physical type which neither wounds nor sickness, unless mortal, could permanently impair, and from the constant handling of their lean, muscular bodies, I came to understand the essential cleanliness and innate nobility of sexual love on its physical side. . . . it was always Roland I was nursing by proxy.[12]

Notably, the emphasis is on the "lean, muscular body" that could embody male virility during and postwar, rather than on the wounds.

While Brittain is careful to constrain her discussion of the relationship between nursing and sexuality within the appropriate narrative of "cleanliness and nobility," her contemporary, Irene Rathbone, is more direct in representing the wounded male body as an object of desire under the control of the nurse: "It gave her a peculiar joy to take hold of a long white arm . . . to wash a muscular young back . . . She was a nurse in uniform, and he was a wounded soldier, the gulf between them was fixed and rigid. And yet across that gulf . . . stretched the faint sweet fingers of sex."[13] The intimate touch that is necessary as a healing ministration at the same time can become the touch of a lover: "the fingers which so swiftly wound the bandage would, she found, if left to themselves, have slipped down to the man's brown cheeks and caressed them."[14] In replacing the injury narrative with the heterosexual erotic, Rathbone brings nurse and wounded soldier into an interdependent relationship that oversteps professional nursing boundaries. In this narrative the healing touch and the erotic touch become so intertwined that they are indistinguishable. In these instances the actual wounds are obscured by "the long white arm" and "muscular young back"; they exist only to provide the opportunity to touch the male body, an action otherwise forbidden. Although Rathbone's *We That Were Young* is fictionalized, it is closely based on her own experiences, and thus can be read as an examination of her own response, or the response of VAD nurses like her, to the wounded men, even if the actual event described above is not strictly factual. Like Brittain, Rathbone is writing postwar, and her representation of nurse and wounded soldier may thus owe something to popular wartime and postwar fiction that was particularly directed toward persuading women of the importance of accepting the wounded as objects of desire. As Jane Potter writes, "the heroes are manly even when and—it can be argued—*because* they are wounded. In fact, wounds are actually sought . . . because they are badges of honour: 'the receipt, stamped and signed upon their bodies, from God and their country.'"[15]

Yet contradictions in Brittain's writings alert us to the conflicting versions of the wounded male body that nurses were compelled to negotiate.[16] Thus while she can acknowledge the erotic potential in nursing wounded men when she revisits her experience more than ten years later, perhaps in an attempt to restore a lost masculinity to these men in the aftermath of the war, in the immediate instance, recorded in her diary and letters, the actuality of her nursing forces her to repudiate her previous fantasy of nursing a wounded Leighton and thus the wound as capital loses its value. By December 1915, there is no romance left in nursing him as a wounded soldier: "I don't want you to get wounded now—not even a little. This War means such a waste of life even when people don't die. And among the few fine examples of humanity that are left whole when it is over I would like to be the one who means so much to me."[17] Thus she rejects the romantic narrative of nurse and wounded soldier-lover and replaces it with the real and terrible damage to the soldier's body. In direct contrast to the erotic narrative of *Testament of Youth*, a letter to Leighton in November 1915 describes her literal immersion in wounds: "One day last week I came away from a really terrible amputation dressing I had been assisting at—with my hands covered with blood and my mind full of a passionate fury at the wickedness of war, and I wished I had never been born."[18]

These conflicting and conflicted representations point to the predicament faced by the woman responding to the wounded soldiers in her care, particularly given her position in the idealized narrative of the heroic wounded soldier and his ministering nurse. On the one hand, the nurse is required to affirm the masculinity of the soldier wounded in the service of his country, an act that carries an erotic undertone; on the other, she is confronted with the emasculating nature of the wounds themselves and with her position as part of the war machine that causes them. Thus even as Brittain romanticizes Leighton's being brought to her hospital, she anticipates Mary Borden's representation of the war as a "conspiracy," also writing to Leighton in October 1915 of the incongruity of:

> the immense importance of the individual and the calm ruthlessness with which hundreds of individuals are mown down . . . Postal Service, A.S.C., R.A.M.C., Taxes, Hospitals etc—all perfectly organized simply to afford the greatest facility to the Science of Death in its noble work of interrupting & nullifying all the other Sciences that make for life.[19]

Yet the dilemma that arises when the nurse confronts her dual role as healer and as part of the war machine that wounds is intensified when we recognize, as she does, the equally important role of restoring dignity to the wounded man, a massive responsibility since nurses' accounts show the burden they carry as proxy for the woman to whom he will return.

When one of American nurse Elizabeth Walker Black's patients in her account *Hospital Heroes* (1919) asks her "do you think she will care for me when I return, a poor mutilé with a changed face," she voices her concern to her reader, "I always worry as to how those wasted bodies and amputated men will be received when they go home."[20] For Black the nurse, as representative of the female gaze that affirms masculinity, must simultaneously acknowledge injury and restore masculinity: "They are more than mangled bodies to be shuddered at, quickly cared for, and passed hurriedly by. Each day men are brought in who have kept the enemy back and saved those behind the lines."[21] Similarly, in an unpublished memoir, Mary Knocker records her response to a young amputee patient: "His greatest sorrow was his determination to release 'his girl' from their engagement, now that he was a cripple. I pointed out that most girls would be proud to marry a war hero like himself, but all of no avail, and he returned to Blighty resolved to sacrifice his happiness."[22] Black's and Knocker's juxtaposing of the "mangled bodies" with the appropriate military courage of these men illustrates the practical lived experience of the dilemma noted earlier. If, as David Morgan notes, "the military represents one of the major sites where direct links between hegemonic masculinities and men's bodies are forged," how can women bear witness to the emasculating results of wounds while at the same time returning dignity to the wounded body?[23]

After nursing at the front for a year, Kate Evelyn Luard probably reflects the experience of most nurses when she states frankly in September 1915 that "there is no form of horror imaginable on any part of the human body that we can't tackle ourselves now."[24] But throughout her letter-journals her representation of injury is constantly qualified by her depiction of the men's courageous stoicism. Thus she can say that "14 hrs a day everyday with these wonderful smashed up soldiers doesn't leave much over at bedtime," but she adds, "they make you feel proud of belonging to the same race."[25] Even while physical damage means they are no longer "whole," Luard restores their masculinity in affirming the extent to which they fulfill a heroic ideal. Her admiration for the men she nurses is undeniably a genuine response to the suffering they are forced to endure, but it is noteworthy that the language she uses constantly affirms the ideals of courage, strength, and endurance that Dawson defines as military virtues that construct an idealized masculinity. In October 1914, working on an ambulance train, she remarks, "They were bleeding faster than we could cope with it; and the agony of getting them off the stretchers . . . is a thing to forget. . . . The outstanding shining thing that hit you in the eye all through was the universal silent pluck of the men."[26] Even though Luard is direct and often unsparing in her writing here, she diverts her own and the reader's gaze from the shared agony of "a thing to forget" to "what hits you in the eye": "the universal pluck of the men."

Her effort to restore to the wounded a masculinity in defiance of their physical mutilation further reminds us of the emotional burden carried by the nurses, since it would seem to arise as much out of a need to retain her own sanity as to affirm their courage. Certainly Luard does not shy away from making direct observations on the war that reveal her anger and frustration. Even in her anonymously published *Diary* (1915) she comments, "One of the most stabbing things in this war is seeing the lines of empty motor ambulances going up to bring down the wrecks who at this moment are sound and fit, and all absolutely ready to be turned into wrecks."[27] Her later collection, *Unknown Warriors* (1930), is more direct. Thus on 24 March 1916 she writes "men are lying out in the cold slush the better to kill each other. Isn't it insane and immoral beyond description?"[28] In May she remarks that "the whole thing seems the same utter waste of life and suffering as it was last May—and the same story of wasted self-sacrifice."[29] Yet these are isolated remarks; for the most part she concentrates on her patients and their endurance. Her desire to highlight the "pluck" of the men is an attempt to pay tribute to their courage in the face of such absurdity, as well, perhaps, as coming out of her own desire to retrieve some affirmation in the face of such suffering, not just for the men but for herself.

Her constant juxtaposing of pain and suffering with heroic endurance, even while she can acknowledge the apparent pointlessness of it, thus points to the problems that attend bearing witness to injury in wartime, and at the same time it shows how the nurse's construction of her relationship with the wounded becomes the means by which she can exert some control over what is essentially an uncontrollable environment. Luard's accounts are striking in their ability to convey very poignantly the experience of nurse and wounded soldier as interdependent, but in achieving this she exchanges the erotic narrative we have seen in Brittain and Rathbone for the culturally sanctioned and thus safe, though equally gendered, nurse-as-mother. In doing so she bears out Christine Hallett's explanation that "nurses used 'familial' relationships with patients to provide comfort while at the same time avoiding the possible dangers of crossing emotional and relational boundaries. They . . . appear to have seen it as part of their duty to avoid both cold professionalism and romantic attachment."[30] It is important to note here that not only was Luard much older than Brittain and Rathbone, but that she was a trained nurse who had served in South Africa; her age and position thus gave her a role unavailable to them. Although, as stated earlier, she finds strength for herself in the stoicism of the "men," she also offers an alternative narrative wherein her patients are helpless "boys" or "lads" or even, at times, infants or babies: "Reggie is worse tonight. He holds out his small hand and says, 'Will you come and sit by me for a little while and hold my hand,'"[31] and comments that "some of them are such infants," referring to one of her patients as "my dear little resuscitated Suffolk boy."[32] When the stoic ideal is removed from both nurse and wounded here, we see the emotional burden of the nurse-mother identity carried by women like her as they watched young men die and wrote what she calls "break-the news-letters" to mothers and wives. In a specific case, when she could have exploited an idealized military masculinity represented by awards, the humanity of the wounded takes precedence; thus writing of RAMC doctor Captain Noel Chavasse, whose extraordinary credentials she lists—VC and Bar, MC, DSO—when he is brought in wounded, for her such symbols of courage are less important than his human yearning: "He tries hard to live, he was going to be married."[33]

The nurses' dilemma in representing their experience then is not only that they are forced to confront conflicting versions of masculinity in the body of the wounded soldier, but that they must negotiate their own gender identities as nurses, whether sisters, lovers, or mothers, in the context of the damaged masculinity of the men they care for. How nurses responded to this dilemma was necessarily influenced by the context in which they wrote and the motives behind their writing.[34] Thus, for example, nurses' memoirs and letters published during the war often detailed the terrible conditions and described the suffering of the wounded but tended to position the harsh conditions against the ideal of sacrifice and the heroic endurance of the medical staff and patients.[35] In particular instances, such as in letters by an American nurse in France, "Mademoiselle Miss," the tone reflects the purpose, here requesting support in the form of supplies: "Gauze, cotton, gloves, and needles all there! Thanks, thanks and God bless you! It's a new year of promise. I believe we *ought* to be joyous no matter if men do try to make it a vale of tears, and the more suffering I see, the more I think so."[36]

In *Hospital Heroes,* apparently mostly written during the war since it ends in medias res with the German advance, Elizabeth Walker Black at times admits that "the feeling of it all being a dreadful nightmare from which we must awaken acted as a narcotic."[37] Yet in the absence of the "narcotic" she must employ a raised rhetoric of sacrifice and service: "I would stagger back at the end of my twenty-four hours to report, with an apron and often a face spattered with blood and mud, and yet a spirit radiant and unweary with the thrill of service."[38] The nurse's intimate engagement with men's wounds marks her physically and emotionally, but the idealization of the nurse's role we see in Black's account does suggest that this arises out of an emotional necessity: without it she could not continue her work. Unlike Vera Brittain, who responds to an amputation by wishing she had never been born, Black finds that "there is regeneration in knowing you can meet the worst and survive."[39] In the immediate situation, with no sense of an ending to the nightmare, nurses seem to need to affirm the ideal of courage and stoicism that they find in the soldiers as a source of emotional strength for themselves, and this need necessarily influences their written response to the wounded. To look beyond the ideal may be psychologically dangerous, but clearly, as we have seen in Brittain's implicating herself in the war machine, nurses were also often troubled by the contradictory nature of their position. Confronting these contradictions may have been difficult or impossible at the personal level, or could not be voiced publicly during the war. Lesley Smith's postwar account, *Four Years out of Life* (1931), however, represents the immersion in hard work and sacrifice as a form of cowardice, calling herself and her fellow nurses by the term given to men who are designated as "embusqués" (shirkers):

> "Of course we'll sign on again," said Gratton acidly. "Are we not the complete *embusqués*? We do our job and it uses up every scrap of time and energy so that we've forgotten there's a war on."
>
> " . . . I feel we're shirking something horribly by just working hard and feeling useful?"[40]

Arguably then, as well as to restore dignity to the wounded body, nurses like Black employ the language of military masculinity to gain some control over the psychological pain caused by what Das calls "the unbearable impotence of sympathy."[41] The interrogation of her position that Smith represents may be too difficult to undertake while actually nursing at the front because it removes a necessary ideological support that keeps the nurse from breaking down. In this interdependent experience, the human connection between nurse and soldier is manifest in the desire to pay tribute not only to his suffering, but also to his ability to endure stoically, a refrain that runs throughout much nurses' writing published during and after the war.

Yet, on the other hand, the lack of a heightened rhetoric in some nurses' private, unpublished diaries or letters suggests that such rhetoric may at times be in response to these accounts as public representations of wartime nursing. While censorship could influence what is not said, as Kate Finzi writes in *Eighteen Months in the War Zone* (1916), "a War Diary published during war time is of necessity much expurgated to meet the demands of the censor,"[42] nurses may also have felt a duty to the men they nursed to maintain the ideologies of stoicism we see in the preceding accounts. Moreover, it is impossible to know how much influence editors and publishers had over the content of wartime memoirs or letter collections or to gauge the extent to which self-censorship may have played a role. It is apparent in Luard's two accounts that there are small but detectable differences between her letter-diaries published during the war and those published later, in that the later collection includes more direct comments about the futility of the war. But at the same time her diaries published anonymously during the war do contain graphic depictions of suffering that could arguably be said to overwhelm the portrayals of stoic endurance. However, without original manuscripts we cannot know whether the difference between the two collections is due to wartime censorship or to Luard's own censoring of her account in the early days of the war.

Unpublished diaries and letters do suggest that the nurses' response to the situation was unavoidably conflicted. Canadian nurse Sophie Hoerner, writing to a friend from a hospital in Etaples, sets her own sense of satisfaction at being there against the nature of her work:

> The patients are so ill in my ward and suffer so terribly that before noon came I thought I would scream myself. I am seeing the grimness of war now and it's awful . . .
>
> We do dressings from nine till twelve, every patient with more than one wound, so terrible I can't describe them . . . but I'm glad I'm here and I am happy.[43]

This letter is representative of Hoerner's telling of her war experience as she writes back to family and friends. She constantly juxtaposes the terrible nature of the wounds and the men's suffering with her own happiness at being there and being able to help. Like other nurses she praises the bravery and cheerfulness of the "Tommies," but does not use the raised rhetoric of sacrifice and stoicism that we have seen in published memoirs. For fellow Canadian nurse Clare Gass there is nothing but suffering unrelieved by any ideology of sacrifice in her private diary description of the wounded from a convoy she receives on 19 June 1915, nor does she remark on her own satisfaction in nursing:

> Some terrible cases, oh so much better dead (one young lad with eyes & nose all gone—one blur of mangled flesh—body whole & sound.) heads shattered to pieces or limbs hanging by a thread of tendons. Oh why must such things be? All are so brave, & yet those who are not badly wounded are so tired of the war, at least those who have been long in the trenches—tired in such a hopeless way.[44]

Although Clare Gass mentions that they are all so brave, she does so in passing; there is no sense that this is in the context of military bravery. Her focus is on the terrible injuries they endure rather than on their courage. Likewise, nurse Mary Brown on a hospital ship receiving wounded from Gallipoli prefers to say nothing than to offset the horror with ideals of heroism: "Before we got breakfast a boat load of wounded came alongside, and all day the boats were bringing them down. We dressed nearly 1,000 . . . We were at it all day had not time to pay attention to the fighting, the whole thing is too ghastly to write about."[45]

Neither Brown nor Gass has the time to take these hurried notes further, but the tone of their terse entries is much closer to accounts by Mary Borden and Ellen La Motte, who confront their position in a nightmare world of fragmented bodies, devoid of meaning, than to the narrative of courage and sacrifice that we find in nurses like Black. Whereas Black and "Mademoiselle Miss" construct their identities in terms of popular gendered ideals of nurse and wounded soldier in spite of the horrifying nature of the conditions, Mary Borden, calling her account of nursing on the western front *The Forbidden Zone* to indicate the multiple transgressions of a woman both placing herself at the front and bearing witness to injury on the male body, enacts for her reader the continual and brutal undermining of a coherent sense of self that is intrinsic to wartime nursing.[46] Intimate physical contact with the wounded, rather than upholding the popular image of the nurse as the ideal of womanhood and the wounded soldier courageous in the face of suffering, is a traumatic shattering of all definitions of gender: "There are no men here so why should I be a woman? There are heads and knees and mangled testicles."[47] As Kaplan writes, "In effect, Borden blurts out the truth: war desexes men and women, and the machine of war truncates, dismembers and atomizes."[48] The popular representations of masculinity and femininity as defined through and in relation to the war-wound are thus revealed to be meaningless.

Both Borden and Ellen La Motte in *The Backwash of War* resist idealized gendered versions of themselves, demonstrating the degree to which they were concerned with subverting the dominant images that supported and perpetuated not just this war, but war as an institution. This involves a systematic interrogation of the relationship between masculinity and femininity and the war. The ideal of the warrior is rejected as a false construction of masculinity, a grotesque conspiracy by government and military that allows countries to exploit and discard the lives of men in the interests of what La Motte calls "Mammon, or the Goddess of Liberty, or Reason as you like."[49] In refusing to participate in the idealized construction of the nurse, Borden and La Motte claim their gaze as one that owns injury, in the sense of Scarry's contention that "war is impossible without the disowning of injury," rather than divert the gaze to a heroic ideal as some nurses feel compelled to do.[50]

While writers like Black uphold the values of a warrior masculinity as they describe the stoicism of their patients and idealize their own roles in relation to it then, Borden and La Motte employ their specific experience as nurses as a legitimate position from which to see and resist war as it is represented and idealized in the image of the warrior. Their recognition of war as a gendering activity brings them to a particular interrogation of and subsequent resistance to the way social constructions of masculinity are instrumental in initiating, supporting, and perpetuating the institution of war. In defining the site from which they see war as peripheral, "the forbidden zone," and the "backwash of war," they give themselves permission to speak of the war through images that resist the dominant rhetoric and define war, as Scarry would much later, as a narrative of the "injury" that is its "main purpose and outcome."[51]

As we have already seen, the recruiting in the opening months of the war in Britain drew on debates about masculinity that were already part of cultural discourse. To quote Nicoletta Gullace:

> As recruiting propaganda evoked prewar concerns [surrounding decadence, effeteness and the potential effeminacy of British youth] "defending the home" came to mean more than rescuing Belgium or preserving the domestic status quo but suggested also the rehabilitation

> of masculinity itself. The belief in the war as somehow "purifying" was intimately tied to the idea that military service would cleanse Britain of the vestiges of *fin de siècle* decadence and produce a regenerate manhood committed to ideas of duty, honor, chivalry, and family.[52]

Central to Borden's and La Motte's resistance to war is a resistance to such constructions of masculine and feminine identities in the service of the war effort; particularly, they subvert a discourse that equates the going to war with the masculine fulfillment in wounding that Leighton writes of before he goes to France, instead presenting war as a systematic process of emasculation.

In her fragment "Moonlight," Borden's uniformed soldier has not been made a man by the war but, rather, deformed by it. His body is taken through a systematic process by which it is harassed by the conditions of war, mutilated by the technology of war, stripped of clothing and dignity by medical staff, and finally stripped of an identity by a system that removes his individuality and when injured defines him only by his injury, "heads and knees and mangled testicles,"[53] and forces him to submit passively to processes of treatment that are represented not as healing but as a further violation of his helpless body. War as a place where a young man can define and test his masculinity through physical hardship, comradeship, and sacrifice is thus revealed to be a hideous deception. Subverting war means rewriting the narrative: the masculinity of the men Borden observes is redefined very emphatically in the context of their domestic lives. In "Moonlight" the false "romance" of war is personified as the harlot pain who is "in the pay of war [and who] amuses herself with the wreckage of men."[54] This perverted sexuality is set against a definition of maleness defined in relation to family. "When they dream of their women and little children, of their mothers and sweethearts, when they dream that they are again clean, normal, real men, filled with a tender and lovely love for women, then she wakes them."[55] More prosaically, Clare Gass similarly observes that her patients define themselves not in terms of the war but of home: "these poor lads, tired in body & spirit, sick of the war . . . aching for their homes & their dear ones."[56]

This emphasis on the domestic challenges the ideal of a masculinity defined by war. In her story "Heroes," La Motte deconstructs the wartime narrative that defines masculinity through abstractions such as courage and sacrifice. "And suddenly she saw that these ideals were imposed from without—that they were compulsory."[57] They do not exist; they are "a state of mind which was not in them, of themselves. Base metal gilded."[58] The imposition of such an ideal she sees as a form of entrapment, even slavery: "[The soldiers] were all harnessed to a great car, a juggernaut, ponderous and crushing, upon which was enthroned Mammon, or the Goddess of Liberty, or Reason, as you like . . . all the Idealists demanded was physical endurance from the mass."[59]

The ideal of bravery that would acknowledge the human potential to rise above this mass endurance is, La Motte reveals in the ironically titled "Pour La Patrie" (For the Fatherland), equally false. Here, when the dying soldier is awarded the Médaille Militaire, "we all knew what it meant. I held the medal before him . . . in its red plush case. It looked cheap, somehow. The exchange didn't seem even."[60] Like the ideals themselves, the medal is a manufactured and hence artificial symbol that is pinned on the body. At the same time La Motte plays on her readers' expectation of the consolation of a heroic narrative. We expect some final recognition of heroism that would redeem the man's lingering and painful death. Instead, she hands the narrative to him: "I was mobilized against my inclination. Now I have won the Médaille Militaire. My Captain won it for me. He made me brave. He had a revolver in his hand."[61] In leaving this image to the very end of the story, La Motte cleverly exploits and then denies her reader's expectations, showing them to be based on the false premise of the heroic ideal. The potential narrative of a courageous act redeeming the conscript's initial unwillingness to fight presupposes the possibility of autonomous action. Instead La Motte exchanges it for a narrative of complete powerlessness.

While La Motte's resistance to the dominant constructions of the ordinary soldier as heroic warrior is revealed in her ironic commentary on a matter-of-fact narrative of events, Mary Borden's resistance is found in her rewriting of the masculine language through which war and the warrior is created. As already mentioned, Borden's resistance to the language of war is equally a resistance to the gendered binaries that place women as nurses and men as soldiers into idealized spheres where each relies on the ideal version of the other as it is represented in popular culture. In order to confront constructions of military masculinity, she must also confront constructions of femininity. The question central to this confrontation—"There are no men here, so how can I be a woman?"—is the site of her resistance to the warrior mythos.[62] War perverts definitions of masculine and feminine. In her fragment entitled "Conspiracy," the domestic imagery implicates women, especially nurses, in the social conspiracy that turns healthy young men with "ruddy faces," "bright eyes," and "strong voices" into the abject: torn and mangled "bundles" that "smell like a corpse," bodies to be disposed of now that their usefulness is over.[63]

Borden emphasizes this process as a given; it leaves no room for dissent: "it is all arranged." Moving between second and third person and from the passive to active voice, she implicates a female audience in the war machine with the extended metaphor of laundering, mending, and finally discarding clothes: "You send your shirts again and again to the laundry . . . you sew up the tears . . . again and again . . . and then you throw them away."[64] Men are materiel, used "so long as they can stand it." Like the "socks and shirts" that are mended "again and again" and then "thrown away," the soldiers are "thrown into the ground."[65] "Do you hear? Do you understand?" she asks at the end. "It is all carefully arranged just as it should be."[66]

Borden's use of the domestic language here retrieves the war story from the language of combat and the discourse of heroism that attends it and offers an alternative language in which to write war. In place of heroic sacrifice men are used and reused "just until they are dead, and then we throw them in the ground."[67] Her systematic collapsing of the dominant wartime rhetoric that persuades men and women to accept the public construction of masculinity and femininity in the cause of "patria" reduces wounding and death in war to a meaningless conspiracy. As in La Motte's writing, the warrior only exists as a rhetorical strategy created to further the war.

As noted previously, Borden's and La Motte's refusal to tell the war story as a narrative of heroism and sacrifice is, at times, shared by other women writing from the war zone, though they are unusual in taking a political position that systematically deconstructs the gendered ideologies that sustain war and belief in war. Examining a range of writings, published and unpublished, we can see that, for the most part, nurses' responses to wartime constructions of masculinity, and of their own identities as nurses, are complex and conflicted. Thus at the personal level, Vera Brittain initially upholds the masculine ideal represented by the wound, but she rejects it as cultural capital once she witnesses the actuality of wounding. For many nurses, adopting a sacrificial narrative both for themselves and for the soldiers they nurse would seem to be a way of coping emotionally with their work. For others, such as Mary Borden and Ellen La Motte, the nursing environment causes them to interrogate and reject not only the construction of a heroic masculinity that serves the state as part of wartime propaganda, but also the representation of the nurses' role as one that perpetuates war. Seen from this perspective, nursing is not a form of care and healing, but rather part of the military machine, complicit in the mutilation and death of men.

Most of the women whose accounts are discussed here do not define their work as a "conspiracy" as directly as Borden and La Motte. Their accounts undeniably reveal conflicting responses, however. At the most private level, for many women the personal involvement with the wounded men in their care is foremost, and it takes precedence over what might be seen as a less human, political response. Moreover, the emotional burden of their own participation in the suffering arguably leads them to look for meaning in ideals of sacrifice both for themselves and the soldier-patients, or at least in the sense of satisfaction they find in their work. Witnessing the men's terrible suffering and death makes it difficult or at times impossible for those caring for them, themselves uninjured, to question the validity of the wounds. The nurses' position thus reflects the larger dilemma for women in wartime: since officially they cannot receive wounds themselves, it is problematic to reject the abstract meaning of the wound as a mark of masculinity; to do so would be to negate the value of the wounded body itself and the sacrifice it represents. If the suffering is meaningless, it may be unbearable.

NOTES

1. Roland Leighton to Vera Brittain, 15 February 1915, in A. Bishop and M. Bostridge, eds., *Letters from a Lost Generation* (London: Little, Brown and Company, 1998), 55.
2. Brittain to Leighton, in Bishop and Bostridge, *Letters*, 76.
3. Brittain to Leighton, unpublished letter, 24 October 1915, Brittain Archives, William Ready Collection, McMaster University.
4. M. Higonnet, ed., *Nurses at the Front: Writing the Wounds of the Great War.* (Boston: Northeastern University Press, 2001), xxxiv.
5. S. Das, *Touch and Intimacy in First World War Literature.* (Cambridge: Cambridge University Press, 2005), 227.
6. Commenting on the wartime song about nurses, "The Rose of No Man's Land," Sharon Ouditt links it to "the popular received image of nurses during the First World War: . . . Eyes uplifted, inwardly grieving, yet externally serene and efficient, she tends to the wounds of the men of her homeland. This stereotype, widely distributed on posters, was as much iconographic as literary. Women had effectively, quickly and cynically been translated into an efficient aspect of wartime propaganda" (*Fighting Forces, Writing Women* (London and New York: Routledge, 1994), 10.
7. G. Dawson, *Soldier Heroes: British Adventure, Empire and the Imagining of Masculinities* (London: Routledge, 1994), 1.
8. T. Tate, *Modernism, History, and the First World War* (Manchester: Manchester University Press, 1998), 94.
9. N. Gullace, *"The Blood of Our Sons": Men, Women, and the Renegotiation of British Citizenship during the Great War* (Houndmills: Palgrave Macmillan, 2002), 38. For an important analysis of the relationship between men and women in the context of men's citizenship as defined in terms of their willingness to go to war, see especially Chapters 2, 4, and 5.
10. J. Bourke, *Dismembering the Male: Men's Bodies, Britain and the Great War* (Chicago: University of Chicago Press, 1996), 31.
11. A. Carden-Coyne. *Reconstructing the Body: Classicism, Modernism, and the First World War* (Oxford: Oxford University Press, 2009), 174.
12. V. Brittain, *Testament of Youth* (London: Virago, 1978), 166
13. I. Rathbone, *We That Were Young* (London: Virago, 1988), 212.
14. Ibid., 155–56.
15. J. Potter, *Boys in Khaki, Girls in Print: Women's Literary Responses to the Great War 1914–1918* (Oxford: Oxford University Press, 2005), 91, quoting R. V. Dolbey, *A Regimental Surgeon in War and Prison* (London: John Murray, 1917), 246.
16. For more general discussion of the contradictory representations of masculinity, femininity, and wartime sexuality, see S. Kingsley Kent, *Making Peace: The Reconstruction of Gender in Interwar Britain* (Princeton, NJ: Princeton University Press, 1993); A. Woollacott, "'Khaki Fever' and Its Control: Gender, Class, Age and Sexual Morality on the British Homefront in the First World War," *Journal of Contemporary History* 29, no. 2 (1994): 325–47; S. Grayzel, *Women's Identities at War: Gender, Motherhood, and Politics in Britain and France during the First World War* (Chapel Hill: University of North Carolina Press, 1999); P. Goodman, *Women, Sexuality and War* (Houndmills: Palgrave Macmillan, 2002).
17. Brittain, unpublished letter, 1 December 1915, Brittain Archives.
18. Brittain, in Bishop and Bostridge, *Letters*, 184.
19. Ibid., 175–76.
20. E. Walker Black, *Hospital Heroes* (New York: Charles Scribner's Sons, 1919), 57.

21. Ibid., 61.
22. M. Knocker, unpublished memoir, "Through Shadows and Sunshine 1914–18," papers of Mary Ethel Cory Knocker (later Love) (1883–1970), Wellcome Trust Library and Archives, GC/258, 60.
23. D. Morgan, "Theatre of War: Combat, the Military, and Masculinities," in *Theorizing Masculinities*, ed. H. Brod and M. Kaufman (Thousand Oaks, CA: Sage Publications, 1994), 168.
24. K. E. Luard, *Unknown Warriors* (London: Chatto and Windus, 1930), 119.
25. Ibid., 172.
26. K. E. Luard (published anonymously), *Diary of a Nursing Sister on the Western Front 1914–1915* (Edinburgh: William Blackwood and Sons, 1915), 89–90.
27. Ibid., 279.
28. Luard, *Warriors*, 44.
29. Ibid., 68.
30. C. Hallett, *Containing Trauma: Nursing Work in the First World War.* (Manchester: Manchester University Press, 2009), 178.
31. Luard, *Warriors*, 74.
32. Ibid., 170.
33. Ibid., 204.
34. For an important discussion of this aspect of war nursing see K. Holmes 'Day Mothers, Night Sisters: World War I nurses and sexuality', in Damousi and Lake eds. *Gender and War: Australians at War in the Twentieth Century* (Cambridge: Cambridge University Press, 1995).
35. For further discussion of such representation, see J. Potter, "'I Alone Am Left to Tell the Tale . . .': Memoirs by Women on Active Service," in Potter, *Boys in Khaki, Girls in Print.*
36. *Mademoiselle Miss, Mademoiselle Miss: Letters from an American Girl Serving with the Rank of Lieutenant in a French Army Hospital at the Front.* (Boston: W.A. Butterfield, 1916), 57.
37. Black, *Hospital Heroes*, 206.
38. Ibid., 219.
39. Ibid., 17.
40. L. Smith, *Four Years out of Life* (Glasgow: Philip Allan, 1931), 67; original italics.
41. Das, *Touch and Intimacy*, 177.
42. K. Finzi, *Eighteen Months in the War Zone: The Record of a Woman's Work on the Western Front* (London: Cassell and Company, 1916), 260.
43. Letter, 2 July 1915, Sophie Hoerner fonds, Library and Archives Canada, Ottawa, Ontario, R2495-0-7-E.
44. C. Gass, *The War Diary of Clare Gass, 1915–1918* (Montreal: McGill Queen's University Press, 2000), 32. Gass's diary was not published until this edition in 2000.
45. M. Brown, unpublished diary, 8 August 1915, Imperial War Museum, 88/7/1.
46. M. Borden, *The Forbidden Zone* (London: Heinemann, 1929) Borden's *The Forbidden Zone* was published in 1929, but she writes in the preface that the sketches, of which "Conspiracy" was one, were written between 1914 and 1918.
47. Borden, *Forbidden Zone*, 60.
48. L. Kaplan, "Deformities of the Great War: The Narratives of Mary Borden and Helen Zenna Smith," *Women and Language* 27, no. 2 (2004): 2.
49. E. La Motte, *The Backwash of War* (New York: G. P. Putnam's Sons, 1934), 24. La Motte's introduction to *The Backwash of War* tells us that it "was first published in the autumn of 1916, and was suppressed in the summer of

1918. . . . From its first appearance, this small book was kept out of England and France. But it did very well in the United States, until we entered the War. Even then, by some slight, it continued to be sold . . . In the summer of 1918, however, something happened . . . The Government, it appeared, did not care for the book" (v–vi).

50. E. Scarry, *The Body in Pain: The Making and Unmaking of the World* (Oxford: Oxford University Press, 1985), 64.
51. Ibid., 80.
52. Gullace, *Blood of Our Sons*, 41.
53. Borden, *Forbidden Zone*, 60.
54. Ibid., 62.
55. Ibid., 63.
56. Gass, Diary, 6 July 1915, 39.
57. La Motte, *Backwash*, 23.
58. Ibid., 23.
59. Ibid., 24.
60. Ibid., 126.
61. Ibid., 131.
62. Borden, *Forbidden Zone*, 60.
63. Ibid., 118.
64. Ibid., 117.
65. Ibid., 117.
66. Ibid., 121–22.
67. Ibid., 117.

8 The Theater of Pain

Observing Mary Borden in *The Forbidden Zone*

Hazel Hutchison

> Mud: and a thin rain coming down to make more mud.
>
> Mud: with scraps of iron lying in it and the straggling fragment of a nation, lolling, hanging about in the mud on the edge of disaster.
>
> It is quiet here. The rain and the mud muffle the voice of the war that is growling beyond the horizon. But if you listen you can hear cataracts of iron pouring down channels in the sodden land, and you feel the earth trembling.[1]

The opening of Mary Borden's war memoir *The Forbidden Zone* (1929) engages the reader's senses in complex and disturbing ways. Ironic in its intensity, immediate in its detachment, and apocalyptic in its absurdity, the narrative voice of this text both relates and embodies the confusion of war. Disconnected impressions of sight, sound, and touch are evoked and then swiftly abandoned—splinters of perception that litter the text without context or coherence, like the wreckage of the battlefield. Only slowly, fragment by fragment, does the reader begin to piece together the landscape of the western front, so familiar to present-day readers through countless books and films, and yet here made raw and offensive once more by the strange bleakness of Borden's language.

The Forbidden Zone is not a well-known text, even among scholars of the First World War. However, those who encounter it quickly recognize its power both as a personal testimony and as a literary artifact. Borden's account of her three-year period as the director of a French military hospital unit was begun while she was serving at the Somme, and sections of it appeared in the *English Review* in August 1917.[2] Although sent to the publisher Collins for consideration in 1917, the full text was silenced by wartime censorship. It was eventually revised, extended, and published in Britain in 1929 and in the US in 1930. Scorned when it first came out for its "ugly images," its "mannerisms," and its "repetitions" of style, and later overlooked by literary critics more interested in the experience of soldier-poets, *The Forbidden Zone* has recently been reprinted and reexamined by readers with an interest in a wider range of wartime perspectives, particularly those of nurses.[3] This remarkable book, with its fearless critique of the militarization of medical care and its poignant awareness of the impact of violence on the physical and emotional life of the individual, gives a vivid insight into the evolving techniques of medical practice in frontline wards, especially as these connect with questions of gender, touch, and trauma. It is usually read in these contexts, when it is read at all.[4] However, Borden's book cannot easily be classified alongside the dozens of eyewitness memoirs written by professional and volunteer nurses about the war, although it flirts continually with the form and tone of such texts. Borden's presentation of herself as an observing innocent in the war zone is undercut by the powerful, unnerving voice with which she delivers her material. This voice is self-consciously literary, starkly modern, and disruptive of the reader's expectations and values. It manipulates perspective and wrong-foots secure moral judgment, making her implied reader—the "you" she addresses on the opening page—a complicit witness to the suffering of the French *poilus* caught in what is presented as a brutal and futile cycle of conflict.

One of the most powerful elements of any text of war—whether poetry, prose, or propaganda—is its capacity to remind us of the powerful relationship between literature and experience. Writing is always more than the simple receptacle of reality. It manipulates responses and shapes patterns of behavior in complex and volatile ways. In the context of a war, words become subtle and dangerous weapons, creating or supporting the deep emotions that drive extreme actions—both for good and for evil. As readers we usually have little trouble accepting that an individual's experience will affect what he or she might write—especially if that experience is traumatic or profound. It is much less easy to quantify how a writer's aesthetic values might define their expectations or determine their behavior, especially in the high-pressure environment of a war zone. But if literature is worth anything, it must be worth something beyond its own boundaries. So, while other approaches to Borden's work have tended to explore how her nursing experience spilled over into her literary creation, this chapter looks at the relationship between art and experience from the opposite perspective. How does literature shape one's experience of conflict and its aftermath? And more specifically: what were the skills and strategies that Borden the writer brought to her task in a military hospital in northern France? These questions lead in turn to further questions about where the functions of writer and nurse intersect and at what point these roles pull apart, revealing the complex tension between life and art.

These issues seem, in Borden's case, to be connected to her use of observation—a process that is also intrinsic to Borden's identity as an American and as a female in the male theater of war. This chapter, therefore, begins by considering how Borden's cultural heritage as a highly literate and affluent American woman shaped her sense of herself as one who watches, and then progresses to examine her use of sight on a number of levels within *The Forbidden Zone*. Observation in this text can mean many things: an uncomprehending survey of the battlefield; a personal engagement with a human drama; an aerial, epic detachment; spying for military purposes; or the intimate and intent process of watching as an element of physical, clinical care. In a number of ways, therefore, *The Forbidden Zone* challenges the idea that seeing is a passive activity, disconnected from the other more tactile senses. In this text, sight, in all its forms, functions as a complex, sometimes dangerous, always powerful, means of experiencing reality.

Borden was born in 1886, the daughter of a Chicago mining and property millionaire. William Borden died when his daughter was eighteen, leaving her a generous inheritance of over ten thousand pounds a year. Mary, known as May to her friends, was educated at home by governesses and later at Vassar College. As a child she yearned to be both a missionary and a writer; as an adult she would fulfill both of these ambitions. While traveling in India with family friends, Borden met a young British missionary, George Douglas Turner, whom she married in 1908. But the marriage was not happy, even when the couple returned to Britain and immersed themselves in the glamorous society of prewar years London and had three daughters. He was quiet and idealistic, while she was extroverted and ambitious. In the years immediately before the First World War, Borden began writing fiction and drama, socialized with figures such as George Bernard Shaw and Ford Madox Hueffer (later Ford), and embarked on a secret affair with the writer and painter Wyndham Lewis, editor of the Vorticist journal *Blast*.

After war broke out in August 1914, Borden left her three small children at home and volunteered, like many other upper-class women, with the French Red Cross. She was posted to a makeshift typhoid hospital in a dilapidated Dunkirk casino, where she was appalled at the lack of organization and resources. Writing after the Second World War, she recalled that hospital as an absurdist nightmare:

> The sick lay helpless under the great tarnished chandeliers of the gaming rooms, the rows of dingy beds were reflected to infinity in the vast gilded mirrors. There were no nurses until we arrived and nothing to nurse with; no feeding cups, no urinals, no bed pans. Even the dying must crawl out of bed and sit on open pails. The wind howled up the beach beyond the great windows, but the stench in the rooms made one vomit.[5]

At this stage, Borden had little nursing or administrative experience, but she did have plenty of money. She wrote to General Joffre, offering to fund and administer a field hospital of one hundred beds under French military command. Borden was told that the French had prepared for twenty-five thousand casualties, but by the end of 1914 half a million men were already sick or wounded. The French army was not in a position to refuse help. So, for the remainder of the war, Borden took responsibility for l'Hôpital

Chirurgical Mobile No. I, a mobile hospital unit staffed by French surgeons, doctors, and orderlies, and British and American nurses. It was stationed initially at Rousbrugge in Belgium, then in the summer of 1916 at Bray-sur-Somme. Later the unit was moved again, during the Nivelle offensive in 1917, but it never left *La Zone Interdite*, the "forbidden zone," behind the front lines, where in theory civilians were not allowed. While at the Somme, Borden met a young English staff officer, Edward Spears, with whom she began a passionate affair. When Turner, who was working as a British army interpreter, discovered the affair, his marriage to Borden finally collapsed. The couple divorced, and Borden married Spears in 1918. After the Conference of Versailles in 1919, they returned to England, where Spears entered politics, later serving as an MP and a diplomat under Winston Churchill, and Borden shaped a successful career writing fiction. Borden's personal wartime narrative reads like a novel—the kind of novel that she herself wrote. Many of her later works such as *Jericho Sands* (1925) and *Sarah Gay* (1931) were shaped by her wartime impressions and desires.[6] Conversely, Borden's experience was also profoundly shaped by her absorption of texts and images, and by her cultural education, which encouraged her to use imaginative strategies and literary tropes to interpret the chaotic stimuli of war. As Christine Hallett notes, First World War nursing memoirs written by trained nurses vary from those composed by volunteers.[7] VADs were usually of a higher social class than professional nurses, and they came to the front with more education and often with unrealistic expectations formed by the sanitized images of recruiting posters and by patriotic romantic novels such as Florence Barclay's *My Heart's Right There* (1915) or Berta Ruck's *Khaki and Kisses* (1915), tales that Jane Potter describes as "part of the public's fantasy investment in the war."[8] Perhaps because of this investment, volunteer nurses were also more likely than their professional colleagues to write emotional and reflective accounts of their experiences, attempting to impose an intellectual or artistic order on their impressions and to reclaim some kind of creative return from the trauma they witnessed. If this was true of many middle-class VADs, it was even more so in the case of Borden, one of the most exclusively and expensively educated women of her generation, well read and well traveled, the product of American wealth and cosmopolitan social polish.

Even before the war began, Borden was playing out a role that had long been a staple of transatlantic fiction: the American heiress unleashed on European society. The novels of Hawthorne, James, Wharton, and many other prewar writers locate this character within the tradition of the American observer in Europe—a figure to whom Europe represented artistic sophistication, culture, and history, but for whom the dislocation of identity set in motion by the collision of these spheres could only end in alienation and dissatisfaction. As Nancy Bentley and Kendall Johnston both show in their researches into cultural consumption, in the late nineteenth and early twentieth century, Europe was primarily a visual experience for Americans, who often made few inroads into social circles, but who went to look at cathedrals, stately homes, and museums in their droves.[9] Lured to travel by exported paintings and photographs, the American tourists' main point of contact with Europe (and with each other in Europe) was the world of the gallery, where they experienced not the life of the Continent, but an artistic interpretation of it, or alternatively the portrait painter's studio or the couture house, where they experienced an artistic interpretation of themselves.

This accent on the visual was also a hallmark of the American literature read by Borden's generation. Thus her expectations of war were shaped through texts very different from the wartime romances of Barclay and Ruck. Borden's own narrative style, with its short sentences and its startling lexical juxtapositions, initially seems to be a text that ruptures language from the conventions of previous literary generations. As Santanu Das remarks: "Here at last is a highly conscious literary modernist."[10] On a closer look, however, many of Borden's virtuoso passages of visual manipulation suggest a felt need for continuity and reinterpretation, a desire to fit her raw experience to ready-made instances of experimental narrative from classic American texts.[11] For example, compare the following passages, both depicting a regiment on the march:

> The regiment was chained to the earth. The men were chained to the ground. They were heavy; they were fastened down. The mass of them jolted along, a dark weight scraping the road. Their flag alone was lifted. It moved fluttering above their heads, tattered and soiled. It was there for an emblem of hope. They ignored it. They did not see it. Long ago they had ceased to regard it.

> When another night came the columns, changed to purple streaks, filed across two pontoon bridges. A glaring fire wine-tinted the waters of the river. Its rays, shining upon the moving masses of troops, brought forth here and there sudden gleams of silver or gold. Upon the other shore a dark and mysterious range of hills was curved against the sky. The insect voices of the night sang solemnly.[12]

The first is the narrative voice of *The Forbidden Zone*, detached and yet detailed, remote and yet lyrical. The second is Stephen Crane's *The Red Badge of Courage* (1895), the only major piece of American war literature to emerge in the twenty years before the First World War. But the tone and narrative formula are so similar that it might be hard to tell on a blind reading to which book each passage belongs. Crane's novella offered his compatriot Borden a stylistic blueprint for a young American author writing about the war, in much the same way as the Civil War itself functioned as the blueprint of modern, industrialized, media-driven warfare.[13] In both texts, the implied observer offers an eerie perspective, distant yet intimate, translating what is happening into a primarily visual event, cataloguing the horror and beauty of war with photographic clarity.

Crane, however, is not Borden's only point of national reference. Walt Whitman's searing impressions of the Civil War also haunt *The Forbidden Zone*, especially its poetry. Whitman's service as a hospital dresser offers Borden a double example for the writer in the war zone: as one who observes and as one who engages with the human consequences of battle. His poems of injury and medical treatment, such as "The Wound-Dresser" and "A March in the Ranks Hard-Prest," create the same sense felt in Borden's work of visual images too strong for full expression, welling up through the plain language of the text. It is often what is omitted that speaks loudest. In both prose and poetry, Borden regularly borrows Whitman's tactic of foregrounding a sentence fragment lacking a principle verb—a tactic that would become a staple of twentieth-century free verse form. For instance, the opening line of her book—"Mud: and a thin rain coming down to make more mud"—syntactically mimics Whitman's opening line, "A march in the ranks hard-prest and the road unknown." In both these examples what is missing from the syntax of the sentence is the verb "to be"—suggesting a problem in both cases with the business of existence. This problem of "who is?" in the text transmutes into the related problem of "who sees?", a problem dramatized for both writers in their use of a high-wire aerial perspective, looking down, birdlike, from a great height on a war-torn nation, a technique that simultaneously places the artist in a privileged, almost godlike vantage point, but also creates an obscuring and distorting distance between speaker and subject, and between speaker and reader. Whitman makes regular use of this perspective in *Drum Taps,* as he does in "Song of Myself."[14] It is also at work in Borden's airborne view of the town under attack in "Bombardment," where the narrative offers a distant view of a distant aircraft bombing a distant town, which is reduced to a flat image by the mechanical viewpoint of the plane itself: "The unconscious map lay spread out beneath it: the wide plain, the long white beach and the sea, lay there exposed to its speeding eye."[15] This distortion of perspective is repeated in the formal properties of Borden's style. In her prose, it manifests itself in clipped sentences and sentence fragments and nonstandard punctuation patterns. In her free verse poems, first published in 1917 when few writers were yet experimenting with such forms, she regularly employs varying line lengths, including the distinctive, long line of Whitman's poetry, curtailed only by the width of the paper on which it is printed, to dramatize the strangeness and confusion of the conflict. This means that, on paper, Borden's poems even look like Whitman's—thus manipulating the reader's experience of vision in yet another way.

In the section entitled "In the Operating Room," Borden goes even further. Here she cuts out the use of narrative perspective altogether, shifting the genre of the text toward drama rather than narrative. She leaves only a disembodied verbal script, in stage-play form, thus inviting the reader to imagine the physical reality of three operations—an amputation, a bullet-ridden lung, and an abdominal shrapnel wound—as the surgeons muse on what they want for dinner:

Nurse: Three knees have come in, two more abdomens, five heads.

Officer (through the window): The *Médecin Inspecteur* will be here in half an hour. The General is coming at two to decorate all amputés.

1st Surgeon: We'll get no lunch to-day, and I'm hungry. There, I call that a very neat amputation.

2nd Surgeon: Three holes stopped in this lung in three minutes by the clock. Pretty quick, eh?

3rd Surgeon: Give me a light, some one. My experience is that if abdomens have to wait more than six hours it's no good. You can't do anything. I hope that chap got the oysters in Amiens! Oysters sound good to me.[16]

This technique is striking, but has, of course, been done before. The theatrical format reprises Herman Melville's use of the same approach in several sections of *Moby Dick*, including Chapter 108—aptly enough also a scene about an amputated leg, where the ship's Carpenter makes Ahab a new stump out of whalebone as they discuss the limits of the human self. In both texts, the lack of a narrating voice is countered by the controlled selection of dialogue, the juxtaposition of characters and events, the "stage" directions, and by the powerful impression of the observing consciousness of the scene. In each example, the effect created is an odd mix of involvement, as though the reader, like the unvoiced observer, is a firsthand witness to events, alongside an oddly comic sense of alienation as the reader is reminded by the visual cues on the page that what they are experiencing is only a text after all.

If it seems fatuous to look at Borden's literary education as a preparation for her experience of the war, it is perhaps wise to remember that for many at the front, this was the only preparation they had. Robert Graves's war memoir *Goodbye to All That* opens with nine chapters offering a detailed account of his early reading and schooling, including his years at Charterhouse School, thus making the disturbing point that a fluency in Classical hexameter verse and (perhaps more usefully) an interest in rock climbing were his most highly developed skills on enlisting as an officer at the age of nineteen.[17] Gertrude Stein recalls that, in her childhood, war was always present through literature, whether the wars of history or of fiction, and so, as she puts it, "there was war all the time."[18] When the First World War broke out, it seemed to her to trigger a sense of recognition of the imagined and vicarious wars already known through text. For some at the front, a literary education could also provide effective if eccentric coping mechanisms. Siegfried Sassoon writes vividly of repeating verse to himself during shell bombardments and of reading to maintain his sense of identity during the endless, impersonal hours of boredom and waiting that army life induced.[19] Thus, Borden's use of the visual tropes of American classic texts in the scenes that she wrote while at the front can be read not merely as a search for shared aesthetic points of reference with her target readership, but also as evidence of how the reading self determines the kinds of experiences we seek out and the ways in which we find significance within these.

For the young American educated in the late nineteenth century, this accent on visual experience was a conscious element not just of literary practice, but also of national identity. Ralph Waldo Emerson's essay "The American Scholar" (1837), a seminal text in the emerging nation's sense of selfhood, categorizes the thinking American man as an observer:

> In silence, in steadiness, in severe abstraction, let him hold by himself; add observation to observation, patient of neglect, patient of reproach; and bide his own time,—happy enough if he can satisfy himself alone that this day he has seen something truly.[20]

In the early stages of the war America itself held observing status, prizing the international neutrality that had been the mainstay of its foreign policy since the end of the Civil War. Borden, like others, seems to have sensed that the war would change the character of American national identity, but the full extent and depth of that change was not yet clear. In the early stages of the war, the gender stereotype that equated observation with a passive femininity became increasingly irksome to those Americans who wished to project an image of their nation as willing and ready to fight. As Mark Van Wienen points out in his studies of American home-front poems during the war, many such poems are preoccupied with asserting the manliness of those in favor of American intervention in the war, and the effeminacy of the pacifist movement.[21] The former president Theodore Roosevelt was a key character in this debate with his desire to purge traits of introspection and diffidence from the American character. True Americans, he wrote, are "resolutely bent upon maintaining our separate, self-respecting, self-reliant national existence"—thus appropriating part of Emerson's agenda while conveniently overlooking his emphasis on detached observation and reflection.[22] This active character, determined, purposefully aggressive, idealistic, and unshakably self-confident, was largely constructed in the shift toward America's military engagement in the war and would have long-reaching effects in the following years.

So, Emerson's desire to "see something truly" was associated with what was by 1914 a conservative sense of American identity, and one that was increasingly connected to a feminine or feminized perspective. Naturally, individuals defied any such categorization. For example, Henry James, whom Roosevelt had dismissed as a womanly deserter of his national identity back in the 1880s, was one of the earliest cultural figures to voice his support for American military engagement in Europe.[23] Conversely, the young Ernest Hemingway, who would become the literary voice of the new, active, self-reliant, masculinized American character, found involvement in the First World War as an ambulance driver in northern Italy, thus viewing the war from the supposedly feminized viewpoint of a noncombatant, medical carer. For Mary Borden, then, the role of the observer was closely tied to her national identity as an American, as well as to her literary antecedents. This observing role was also, increasingly, perceived as a role for women, the passive complement to masculine action and engagement, and it would define both her role in the hospital unit and her artistic portrayal of this. The figure of the watching woman is a powerful one in *The Forbidden Zone*, although the gender politics of who is watching whom are continually disrupted and renegotiated within this text.

The role of the nurse in war highlights many feminized qualities widely perceived in the early twentieth century as essentialist and immutable: empathy, responsiveness, patience, and nurture. So natural did the equation of women with nursing seem at the outbreak of the First World War that most people found it impossible to imagine them participating in any other way.[24] Borden appears to have accepted this nurturing role, at least to a certain extent. As Higonnet notes, for Borden, "nursing must be a kind of resistance to the physical and spiritual destruction of the war."[25] This resistance is evident at several points in *The Forbidden Zone*; for example, in her description of the new process of triage, in which the hopeless cases were sorted out from those who had a chance of survival. Borden portrays this as a practice that relied on the close observation of her patients:

> It was my business to sort out the nearly dying from the dying. I was there to sort them out and tell how fast life was ebbing in them. Life was leaking away from all of them; but with some there was no hurry, with others it was a case of minutes. It was my business to create a counter-wave of life, to create the flow against the ebb. It was like a tug of war with the tide.[26]

In this situation her judgment routinely relies on the use of touch, checking the patient's heart rate and temperature, but this level of intimacy was not always possible: "Sometimes there was no time to read the ticket or touch the pulse. . . . I could look down over the rough forms that covered the floor and pick out at a distance this one and that one. I had been doing this for two years, and had learned to read the signs."[27] Here, observation, even looking down from a distance as her narrative does elsewhere, carries out that female, life-giving role—but it is no longer passive. It is the exercise of her power over her patients, quite literally the power of life and death, and one that, aptly enough, takes the form of reading. The ability to decode linguistic signs and concepts translates into a sensitivity to, and an ability to shape, human events. She can read the physical features of the men as readily as she can read the tickets by which they are labeled. Given Borden's apparent confidence in her visual skills it is perhaps ironic that this chapter carries the title "Blind," partly in reference to the blinded soldier waiting for treatment who can neither see nor hear what is happening around him and therefore fears that he is alone, but also as a suggestion of the blind figure of fate that Borden has become. In this chapter she deals out death as well as life, giving the fatal double dose of morphine that the surgeon prescribes for a hopelessly wounded man. The surgeon tells her: "In cases like this, if I am not about, give morphine; enough, you understand?"[28] The text does not answer the unspoken question: enough for what?

This tacit agreement that the soldier is better off dead defies medical protocol. Nevertheless, it seems less brutal than the forced complicity demanded of the nurse in the destructive process of war. Borden herself articulates this contradiction in the section "Rosa," where the nurses are expected to nurse back to health a soldier who has attempted to commit suicide, in order that he can be court-martialed and shot as a deserter.[29] Determined to die, the man tears off his bandages night after night, and day after day the nurses replace them, until Borden intervenes, instructing the night nurse not to re-dress the wound: "She looked at me a minute hesitating. She was highly trained. Her traditions, her professional conscience, the honor of her calling loomed for a moment before her, then her eyes lighted. 'All right', she said."[30] As with the double dose of morphine, there is an understanding by the nurses that in such a circumstance death is the best care they can give. But here the power of the female nurse over the passive patient demonstrates the failure of the conventional sexual hierarchy, especially as the nurses' defiance deliberately undercuts the male chain of command of army regulations, which would have them restore the soldier's physical self at the expense of his emotional self—only to destroy him all over again. In this story, the problem of gender is neatly highlighted by Borden's strategy of referring to the soldier as "Rosa," the woman's name he calls out repeatedly, the name of the woman who is, Borden guesses, the real cause of his wish to die. Freedman interprets Borden's disruption of gender as a means for cutting through the deadwood of social convention and reducing figures to physical, material creatures. In so doing, Freedman argues, Borden offers herself to the reader as a bridge between the chaotic world of the field hospital and the world of the reader, situating herself "in a sequestered zone between the home front and the front line, as well as between traditionally gendered roles." In this chaotic world, Freedman concludes, "Gender itself has been wounded."[31] In "Moonlight" Borden articulates the impact on her own sense of female identity of repeatedly witnessing and participating in this process:

> There are no men here, so why should I be a woman? There are heads and knees and mangled testicles. There are chests with holes as big as your fist, and pulpy thighs, shapeless; and stumps where legs once were fastened. There are eyes—eyes of sick dogs, sick cats, blind eyes, eyes

> of delirium; and mouths that cannot articulate; and parts of faces—the nose gone, or the jaw. There are these things, but no men; so how could I be a woman here and not die of it?[32]

The body of gender is not merely wounded, but dismembered, its body parts strewn around the hospital site like those of a shell-blast victim. What remains is not only nongendered, but almost inhuman, with the "eyes of sick dogs, sick cats." Eyes are important in *The Forbidden Zone*, and the eyes of the patients in this section create yet another problem for Borden. The nurse who watches is in turn observed by her patients—at least by those patients who still can watch. *The Forbidden Zone*, with its multiple points of view and its shifts from first-person to third-person narrative, shows an awareness of Borden's sense of herself not just as an observer, but also as an object of observation. For example, the section "The Regiment" appears to be a reworking of the ceremony in which Borden was awarded her *Croix de Guerre* by General Pétain in June 1917.[33] However, in the text, again narrated from a point of remote observation, she appears as a strangely exotic figure in white watched by the men in the square. She is both "a teasing current of delight touching the officers" and "a strange fantastic thing, like a white peacock" to the people of the town. The wise old men of the regiment are too tired to bother about such a creature.[34]

One of the series of unpublished sonnets that Borden wrote to Spears at the height of their affair in 1917 also deals explicitly with her sense of being watched as she works:

> The patient wounded in their narrow beds
> Welcome me and smile as I go by
> Down the long wooden buildings where they lie
> Wan weary rows of helpless haggard heads—
> Mysterious burning eyes that seem to gaze
> From a great distance, gaze, but do not know
> Why they are glad to see me come and go.
> Sometimes with feeble hands as in a daze
> They beckon me, poor things that vaguely grope
> Out of great darkness toward a distant light;
> And from the unknown woman dressed in white
> They seem in some strange way to gather hope—
> They do not know that in this shadowed place
> It is your light they see upon my face.[35]

Carol Acton, Santanu Das, and Max Saunders all note that the position of the noncombatant witness in the war zone is complicated by the politics of desire set in motion by the very act of watching—by the power of the "gaze."[36] This term is adapted from film theory, where rather than characterizing observation as a passive, feminized activity, Laura Mulvey ascribes a masculine quality to the process of watching. For Mulvey, the gaze of the camera is associated with the (usually) male gaze of the director, who forces the audience to look at things as a man does, thereby objectifying and effacing the female figure.[37] Something similar appears to be happening in Borden's poem through the insistent gaze of the wounded patients, although it is perhaps inevitable that watching as a form of agency and assertion should be central to any literature written in a war zone, where spying and keeping lookout are essential parts of battle planning. As Caroline Brothers observes, the use of photography as both a military and propaganda tool, which was pioneered in the First World War, has been developed to such an extent "that sight itself has become a weapon in combat, beginning even to overtake conventional armor in military and strategic importance."[38] *The Forbidden Zone* regularly features military watchers of different types, including spy-planes, the observation balloon tethered near the hospital, or the watching guards at the Belgian army HQ. The male status of these guards, however, does not protect them from the interpretative gaze of the narrator and the reader. Watched as well as watching, it is the eyes of these men that betray the futility of their masculine, soldierly role. "You can read on their heavy jowls," Borden writes, "in their stupefied, patient, hopeless eyes, how boring it is to be a hero."[39]

In Borden's sonnet, the speaker's observation of the patients as helpless and haggard is met by their gaze, a gaze that like the narrative voice of *The Forbidden Zone* at times, is "from a great distance." The gaze is also unknowing, but it is not without a kind of agency. Through it the patients seem "in some strange way to gather hope," but it also has the effect, like Mulvey's cinematic gaze of the male director/spectator, of stripping the speaker of her identity. As in "The Regiment," she becomes "the unknown woman dressed in white," an empty figure, a blank page. However, the two-line "turn" at the end of the poem provides a further twist to the politics of vision in this sonnet. The speaker reveals the secret that the patients have not seen her at all, but have only seen something of the absent male lover reflected in her face, as though she were the moon casting the sun's light. Ultimately, the gaze of the patients cannot contain or objectify the woman in white, who escapes out of the poem to assume the position of speaker.

The sense of remoteness at the heart of the patient–nurse relationship in "The Patient Wounded" hints at a deeper irony in the gender politics of Borden's experience of watching. Despite her willingness to assume the life-giving, caring female role stereotypically associated with nursing that she demonstrates in "Blind," the truth must have been that Borden had little time to do very much hands-on nurturing. This sonnet gives the impression of a rather quick stroll around the wards, rather than the intimate encounters of touch and conversation that are usually associated with the ideal of nursing practice. Borden did regularly take her turn on the wards, but her main role in the hospital was that of *Directrice*. Numbers of patients and staff clearly varied, but however you analyze them they are remarkable. In Belgium in 1915 Borden's hospital originally had a modest 160 beds to twelve nurses, whereas the larger operation she oversaw in the Somme had, according to Spears, sometimes as many as three thousand patients.[40] Eighty percent of the men who made it as far as Borden's hospital survived. After the move to Bray-sur-Somme in 1916, Borden was forbidden to take British or American nurses back into the French militarized zone and had to rely on a ludicrously small number of French nurses, sometimes as few as twelve, although this rose to fifty by the end of the conflict.[41] In practice, this must have meant a huge reliance on male orderlies, "the old ones," as Borden calls them, who carried out much of the handling of the patients, the cutting away of uniforms, the washing and dressing of wounds. The surgeons and doctors also were male, as were most of the ambulance drivers. So, while these carers performed what can be read as "female" roles, it would certainly be a mistake to think of the hospital as predominantly a female zone. In Borden's case, therefore, her job as *Directrice* of the hospital must have entailed spending the majority of her time employed in yet another kind of observation, this time for the purposes of managing her staff and resources. Indeed this is the sense that one gets of her from reading La Motte's account of her time with Borden's unit in Belgium, *The Backwash of War*, where Borden appears in "her immaculate starched skirts," cool and capable, if a little remote, dropping in to keep an eye on things.[42] This appropriation of the *Directrice* as a persona within La Motte's text adds further level of observational complexity to Borden's experience. The intense to-and-fro of visual sexual politics within the hospital—women watching men watching women—is reproduced, multiplied, and ultimately diffused by the sense of Borden being exposed to the observation and interpretation of another woman. She is then in turn open to the observation and interpretation of the readers of both texts, male and female. In this crowded theater of war, there are a great many people watching from many different viewpoints—a situation that, as Margaret Higonnet points out elsewhere in this volume, disrupts any attempt at cohesion in reportage of frontline experiences.

If all of this suggests that Borden was intent on a highly sophisticated and progressive manipulation of the performative nature of gender roles, one should note that her letters to Spears, in which her love poems were both literally and conceptually folded, were often strikingly conventional and heavily reliant on literary tropes. She addresses him as a medieval knight, a commander, a Viking, as "the future King of Europe," while she appears as a "little goddess," as "a little frail thing," and as "a creature to be protected."[43] And she gives plenty of other evidence elsewhere that her gender politics are not as militant as many of her critics might like to believe. Beyond the war zone, Borden's tussle with the stereotypes of gender was complex and contradictory. Radical and permissive in many areas such as divorce, contraception, votes, and jobs for women, she nevertheless displays some nostalgia for more conservative patterns of interaction between the sexes, especially within the family. Likewise, within *The Forbidden Zone*, Borden's conflicting perspectives on gender roles lie across each other, often within the same passage or poem, creating a complex web of contradictory positions and ideas, similar to the mesh of multiple lines of observation drawn by the watchers and watched within the text. And this, in turn, replicates a wider pattern of contradictory responses to the war as a whole. Sandra Gilbert describes the First World War as "a festival of female misrule" that prompted the "collapse of a traditional social structure" by providing women with social and sexual liberation through their newfound national usefulness and their access to well-paid employment, and she calls attention to the many memoirs that contrast women's sense of "genteel immobilization with the exhilaration of military mobility." [44] However, the work of a very wide range of female writers, across national divides, including H. D., Edith Bagnold, Vera Brittain, Maud Mortimer, and Virginia Woolf, shows that the initial sense of purpose and liberation experienced by mobilized women often gave way to more nuanced responses of dismay, horror, and resignation—suggesting that their emotional experience was not so very different from that of mobilized men. Thus, as Trudi Tate points out, "gender is only one aspect of subjectivity and of writing," and there is a danger in focusing on this theme as "a final point of inquiry" as though the First World War was fought over this issue.[45]

Borden's visual politics are complex. They are shaped and guided by the very conventions of gender and nationality that they attempt to disrupt, making it impossible to map the patterns of such themes neatly within her work or to reduce her complex responses to a single position—which is perhaps why *The Forbidden Zone* can claim to be a great text. Indeed, Borden herself is self-consciously aware of the dangers and difficulties of attempting to generate overarching conclusions about anything as chaotic as war. In the preface to the book, she offers a defense of her disjointed and unstable narrative method: "To those who find these fragments confused, I would say that they are fragments of a great confusion. Any attempt to reduce them to order would require artifice on my part and would falsify them." This is a slightly disingenuous statement at the beginning of one of the most stylized accounts of the war, one that is profoundly artificial in the sense of being art. However, Borden shows her awareness here that writing about reality is a complicated business, one not always best served by the attempt to produce an objective linear account. Indeed, the beauty and the power of *The Forbidden Zone* as a literary text lie in its poetic correlation between form and content; the conflicting narrative perspectives and genres parallel the sensual and moral disruption the text itself describes. Even so, Borden's preface acknowledges that this text will always remain inadequate for those who experienced the reality of the war, those who know "all the rest that can never be written." *The Forbidden Zone* therefore offers a sophisticated consideration of the important, yet limited, role of the witness-participant in the war zone, a figure who does offer some kind of bridge between the front line and the home front, as Freedman asserts, but one who can only do so by acknowledging the impossibility of ever fully reaching across this gap. The writer, therefore, like the nurse, finds that there is often little they can do in the war zone other than watch. Yet, as *The Forbidden Zone* demonstrates, watching is not a simple process, but a complex means of interaction, one that can carry a bewildering range of emotions and intentions between people. Ultimately, Borden shows us that there is something profoundly human, even redemptive, in the act of offering one's attention to the spectacle of individual suffering in the midst of such large-scale destruction.

ACKNOWLEDGMENT

I thank Duff Hart Davis for his generosity in giving permission to publish in full "The Patient Wounded" by Mary Borden.

NOTES

1. Borden, *The Forbidden Zone*, 1.
2. M. Borden-Turner, "At the Somme," *English Review* (August 1917): 97–102, 341–487.
3. *The Times Literary Supplement* (5 December 1929): 1030. Borden, *The Forbidden Zone*. Sections of *The Forbidden Zone* and La Motte, *Backwash*, are reprinted in Higonnet, *Nurses at the Front*.
4. Das, "The Impotence of Sympathy"; A. Freedman, "Mary Borden's Forbidden Zone: Women's Writing from No-Man's Land," *Modernism/Modernity* 9, no. 1 (2002): 109–24; Kaplan, "Deformities of the Great War"; M. Gordon Krob, "Commentary on 'Rosa,'" *Academic Medicine: The Journal of the Association of American Medical Colleges* 77, no. 7 (2002): 710–11.
5. M. Borden, *Journey down a Blind Alley* (London: Hutchinson, 1946), 8.
6. M. Borden, *Jericho Sands* (London: Heinemann, 1925). M. Borden, *Sarah Gay* (London: Heinemann, 1931).
7. "Texts produced by trained professionals were very different from those of volunteers. The former tend to be factual and pragmatic, whereas the latter are often reflective and sometimes assertively opinionated. Because volunteer nurses (VADs) were more likely to be from a higher social status than trained nurses, their writings were attributed a higher intrinsic value in their own time, and are therefore more likely to have been preserved and, indeed, published" (Hallett, "The Personal Writings of First World War Nurses," 321). Santanu Das also addresses the question of class in nursing in *Touch and Intimacy*, 189.
8. Potter, *Boys in Khaki, Girls in Print*, 91. F. Barclay, *My Heart's Right There* (New York and London: G. P. Putnam's Sons, 1915). B. Ruck, *Khaki and Kisses* (London: Hutchinson, 1915).
9. N. Bentley, "Museum Realism," in *Cambridge History of American Literature* (Cambridge: Cambridge University Press, 2005), 3:65–106; K. Johnson, *Henry James and the Visual* (Cambridge: Cambridge University Press, 2007).
10. Das, *Touch and Intimacy*, 220.

11. In *The American Classics,* Denis Donoghue contests T. S. Eliot's definition of a classic as a work of cultural, linguistic, and authorial maturity. Donoghue bestows classic status on *The Scarlet Letter, Moby Dick, Leaves of Grass, Walden,* and *Huckleberry Finn* for their ability to offer American readers "a shared cultural experience" and to "put in question the otherwise facile ideology of individualism on which American culture complacently prides itself"—a set of criteria that considerably broadens the field. D. Donoghue, *The American Classics: A Personal Essay* (New Haven, CT: Yale University Press, 2005), 19.
12. Borden, *The Forbidden Zone*, 29; S. Crane, *The Red Badge of Courage* (Oxford: Oxford University Press, 1995 [1895]), 19.
13. For a fuller discussion of the impact of photography and newspaper coverage on the American Civil War, see B. Harris, *Blue and Gray in Black and White: Newspapers in the American Civil War* (Washington, DC: Brassey's, 2000); and H. Dicken Garcia and G. Dell'Orto, *Hated Ideas and the American Civil War Press* (Spokane: Marquette Books, 2007).
14. For example, see "From Paumanok Starting I Fly Like a Bird" and "Bivouac on a Mountain Side," W. Whitman, *Leaves of Grass*, ed. S. Bradley (New York: Norton, 1973), 284, 300.
15. Borden, *The Forbidden Zone*, 5.
16. Ibid., 135.
17. Graves, *Goodbye to All That*, 36–68.
18. G. Stein, *Wars I Have Seen* (London: Brilliance Books, 1984 [1945]), 7.
19. Ironically, it was no great work of literature that repeated in Sassoon's mind under bombardment, but an incomplete advertisement slogan: "They come as a boon and a blessing to men / The Something, the Owl and the Waverley Pen"; see S. Sassoon, *Memoirs of an Infantry Officer* (London: Faber and Faber, 2000 [1930]), 50.
20. R. Waldo Emerson, "The American Scholar" (1837), in *Collected Works*, 5 vols., ed. R. E. Spiller and A. Ferguson (Cambridge, MA: Harvard University Press, 1973), 1:63.
21. M. Van Wienen, *Partisans and Poets: The Political Work of American Poetry in the Great War* (Cambridge: Cambridge University Press, 1997), 58–59.
22. T. Roosevelt, "Foreword," in *One Hundred Percent American*, ed. A. Squires (New York: George H. Doran, 1918), viii.
23. For a full account of James and Roosevelt's complex and sometimes hostile relationship, see P. Horne, "Henry James and 'The Forces of Violence': On the Track of 'Big Game' in 'The Jolly Corner,'" *Henry James Review* 27, no. 3 (2006): 237–47; P. Horne, "Reinstated: James in Roosevelt's Washington," *Cambridge Quarterly* 37, no. 1 (2008): 47–63.
24. Jenny Gould writes that "when war broke out, the only military sphere in which women were accepted was their traditional role of caring for the sick and wounded," while the idea of them taking part in battle was generally seen as "disturbing and offensive." J. Gould, "Women's Military Services in First World War Britain," in *Behind the Lines: Gender and the Two World Wars*, ed. M. Higonnet et al. (New Haven, CT: Yale University Press, 1987), 116, 117.
25. Higonnet, *Nurses at the Front*, xx.
26. Borden, *The Forbidden Zone*, 143.
27. Ibid., 145.
28. Ibid., 140.
29. La Motte describes what appears to be the same set of events in "Heroes" in *Backwash*, 15–24.
30. Ibid., 105.

31. Freedman, "Mary Borden's Forbidden Zone," 121.
32. Borden, *The Forbidden Zone*, 60.
33. For details of Borden's awards from the French government, see Spears's lengthy correspondence from 1918 on the Foreign Office's reluctance to grant Royal Assent for Borden's award of the Legion of Honor. Churchill College Archive, Cambridge, SPRS 11/2/2.
34. Borden, *The Forbidden Zone*, 35.
35. MB to ES, 17 April 1917, Churchill College. Used by permission of Duff Hart-Davis.
36. C. Acton, "Diverting the Gaze: The Unseen Text in Women's War Writing," *College Literature* 31, no. 2 (2004) 53–79; Das, *Touch and Intimacy*, 220–25; M. Saunders, "War Literature, Bearing Witness, and the Problem of Sacralization: Trauma and Desire in the Writing of Mary Borden and Others," in *Memories and Representations of War: The Case of World War I and World War II*, ed. E. Lamberti and V. Fortunati (Amsterdam: Rodopi, 2009), 177–192.
37. L. Mulvey, "Visual Pleasure and Narrative Cinema," *Screen* 16, no. 3 (1973): 6–18. For a discussion of the value of Mulvey's theory and alternative visual strategies for analyzing sexual difference in the context of war writing, see Tate, *Modernism*, 97–102.
38. C. Brothers, *War and Photography: A Cultural History* (London: Routledge, 1997), 1.
39. Borden, *The Forbidden Zone*, 2.
40. Edward Spears to Leroy Lewis, 17 June 1918, Churchill College.
41. Borden, *Journey down a Blind Alley*, 9.
42. Borden, *The Backwash of War*, 202.
43. MB to ELS, 11 September 1917 and 18 August 1917.
44. S. Gilbert, "Soldier's Heart: Literary Men, Literary Women, and the Great War," in *Behind the Lines: Gender and The Two World Wars*, ed. M. Higonnet et al (New Haven, CT: Yale University Press, 1987), 197–226, 212 and 214.
45. Tate, *Modernism*, 4–5.

9 Cubist Vision in Nursing Accounts

Margaret R. Higonnet

The souls that sleep shall wake again,
And blinded eyes must learn to see.

(Vera Brittain, "August 1914")[1]

The multiplication of the means of observation, both by deploying all the senses and by enhancing observation through technological innovation, is fundamental to the modern practice of medicine. Nurses' descriptions of their work in First World War literature underscore the importance of exploiting every source of information, or what Michel Foucault calls the "plurisensorial structure" of perception enhanced by discoveries such as Roentgen's X-rays or Laennec's stethoscope.[2] The nurse listens not only to whistlings, cracklings, and rumblings, but also with an ear attuned to the quality of a voice or its unconscious ravings, as André Breton did when he was an orderly at the Val de Grâce military hospital in Paris.[3] Another contributing sense would be the touch—which as Santanu Das has noted, captures fever, pulse, and distension.[4] A stench may be a telltale sign of gas gangrene. Urine may be seen, smelled, even tasted. Yet, as Foucault argues, the "visible" most broadly remains the dominant sense. In 1914–1918, the medical gaze holds particular significance in nurses' narratives, in part because of the contributions of Marie Curie to radiology as an instrument of wartime medicine. In her book *La Radiologie et la guerre* (Radiology and War, 1921), Curie laid out the importance of X-rays for the surgeon who sought to locate shrapnel or a broken bone. The successful tactic, she explained, was the "double image"—two X-rays taken at different angles.[5] The basic principle of triangulation, together with the visual penetration through the opacity of the body, pinpoints the medical target before the surgical cut opens up the body. Foucault describes this structure as one of "invisible visibility." The image as symptom offers knowledge: what is hidden becomes transparent, revealing truth.[6] As Foucault notes, the body becomes a text to be read, and its symptoms unveil maladies that are not only pathological, but social and moral. Enhanced modes of medical vision may have prepared nurses to exploit changing artistic modes of visual representation. Furthermore, the high incidence of facial wounds caused by gas or shells that blinded soldiers in 1914–1918 focused social anxieties on the patient's own gaze as a vulnerable and ambiguous instrument of communication and knowledge.

My focus here will therefore be on a multiplication of perceptions in the pursuit of new understanding that we find in nurses' writings about the Great War, both as theme and as narrative strategy. I will argue that the multiplication of angles of perception operates at many levels. As I have shown elsewhere, the juxtaposition of word and image in women's wartime scrapbooks can become a compound form of stereoscopic memoir that I call a "photo-text." [7] Florence Farmborough, for example, publishes in two different media (a diary with a few photographs and a photographic album with a few explanations), in order to represent what she observes—both verbally and visually. While I see these as a compound narrative, subject to editorial intervention for economic reasons, Clare Tylee has compared Farmborough's diary-memoir *Nurse at the Russian Front* to her album of photographs, *Russian Album*, speculating that Farmborough's photographs aimed to salvage dignity in the face of degradation that defeated speech.[8] Double narratives, in short, are subject to interpretation, just as single narratives are.

What I want to suggest is that nursing texts about the First World War can be read at the intersection of three disciplines, since their strategies bring to bear the concerns of medical history, historical testimony, and literary artistry. Here I focus on narrative experiments with voice, with the splitting of characters, and with a dialectic exchange of gazes between nurse-narrator and soldier-patient. In classic examples of irony, the nurse-narrator may offer two very different images of the same person. She may present the tension between two nurses with different attitudes; she may ironically split the narrative voice itself—a tactic that Jane Marcus has observed in Evadne Price's novel *Not So Quiet . . .* (1930), which is narrated in the first-person voice of a VAD worker. Both Claire Tylee and Marcus suggest that writers use the voice of a nurse ironically to juxtapose their "anesthetized" or suppressed emotions with private revelations, creating an "illusion of multiple voices."[9] In the visual realm, Jean Gallagher's study, *The World Wars through the Female Gaze*, finds that women's war photography presents a self-conscious model of "fragmented or indirect visual apprehension" that has been obstructed by blockages in vision, to suggest censorship and resistance.[10] Such verbal and visual strategies converge, I propose, with the modernist breakup of perspective at the same time that they drive toward an epistemology that seeks out a more profound version of "the truth." My path diverges from that of Eric Leed, who in *No Man's Land* (1979) notes a "fragmentation of vision," especially through the constriction of vision in the trench, and who therefore asserts that for soldiers hearing became "more important than vision as an index of what was real and threatening."[11] Alternatively, Das has explored the rich haptic features of nursing texts resistant to verbalization, whose tactile details were long overlooked. While undoubtedly these other senses do play important roles in many medical narratives, my focus here will be on vision and its deployment ultimately to raise questions about moral perspective.

Experiments with fractured perspective had become familiar by 1914; they had already been assimilated to the representation of war. Most spectacularly, cubist artists in the circle around Picasso, Braque, and Gertrude Stein had broken by 1909 with a unified perspective and developed a technique of capturing multiple planes, as if from multiple angles or at successive points in time. David Cottington has pointed out that in 1912, an important year of cubist innovations, Picasso embarked on *papiers collés*, following Braque's collage techniques, and incorporated "newspaper reports of the progress of the war in the Balkans."[12] That conjunction, he argues, shows the interplay between "history" and artworks, as well as the artistic appropriation of "popular" materials. He draws on Patricia Dee Leighten's argument that Picasso's anarchist background led to anti-war citations or collage clippings of political reports, such as a story about a socialist demonstration in Paris against the Balkan War. Leighten notes that Picasso "meticulously cut and pasted to preserve legibility" newspaper clippings that "heralded the approach of World War I and the anarchist and socialist response."[13] More than half of the clippings he included in 1912–1914 drew on such reports, foreshadowing a European war; he pasted his clippings onto images that set these debates in the context of cafés where artists congregated to engage in their political debates. We might add that the layered effects of collage were akin to the cubist fascination with masks, such as the Fang masks collected by Derain and Vlaminck and painted in *Les Demoiselles d'Avignon* (1907) by Picasso. In a troubling augury of the war to come, whose impact would last for decades, many of these masks were marked by scarification.

When Gertrude Stein invited nurses Mary Borden and Ellen La Motte during the war to her home, where works by Picasso and other artists from her circle were on display, they had an opportunity to connect such visual experimentation with Stein's verbal experiments and with their own knowledge of medical practices of visualization. The deconstruction of the body was central to these practices, although I will argue here that social anatomy is as central to wartime writing as is physiological anatomy. Marcel Duchamp's *Nude Descending a Staircase, No. 2* (1912) used the splitting up of the body to lay bare the nude in a new way and to propel a static image into motion through space, to animate the frozen pose, in what we might consider a dynamic perspectival anatomy rather than a physical one. This scandalous painting has also been read as combining mechanistic facets with the dynamic forms of Futurism. Such combinatory esthetics can be interpreted as a fusion of different disciplines. Thus Mark Antliff and Patricia Leighten argue in *Cubism and Culture* that X-rays as well as Henri Bergson's theories of perception influenced cubist experiments and thus brought the connections among philosophy, medicine, and artistic representation full circle.[14] If multiple X-ray images open up access to breaks in a bone or to alien bodies such as shrapnel, experimentally layered narrative perspectives may expose breaks and incoherence in social logic.

Going back deeper into the middle of the nineteenth century (roughly the 1860s), the double image of the stereoscope had served domestic entertainment. During the war it served military analyses of aerial photographs taken in stroboscopic shots. That doubling of the image aimed to produce an illusion of depth, or an approximation of "the real," converting the flat image through our binocular vision into a three-dimensional image. Inevitably, the stereoscope fascinated thinkers because it reminded them that such illusionistic images are a mental product, not a sensory fact. German novelist Ernst Jünger describes "stereoscopic" vision as one that permits the soldier to view himself as both subject and object, thereby fusing objective and subjective representation.[15] What I am calling attention to here in modernist nursing accounts, however, differs from stereoscopy, in that the divergent angles often underscore a rupture in the familiar conception of "the real," rather than bring together perspectives to join in an illusion of coherence. The near repetition esthetically serves a modernist disjunction. Politically it satirizes an ideological quest for a seamless, intangible truth. An alternative interpretation of stereoscopy might be drawn from yet another discipline: ethnography. At the turn of the century, anthropologists had begun to recognize the significance of autoethnography to the ethnographic gaze, alternating between the positions of controlling scientific subject and object of one's own corrective gaze in order to achieve a secondary mode of control and self-reflexive objectivity. We can perhaps see this in Dr. W. H. R. Rivers's double-blind experiments on himself as psychologist as well as anthropologist. But rather than the disciplinary equilibrium sought by Rivers in his experiments and in his treatment of war-shocked patients at Craiglockhart, a disturbing turn in the nurse-narrator's representation of the nurse-figure and her internal debates, as well as of the patient under multiple gazes, may lead us toward a destabilizing of medical authority. Likewise, the reverse gaze of the patient complicates claims of authority and traditional ethnography.

The quest for truth in the shifting and chaotic conditions of war drives the ironic ambiguities of the "invisible visibility" in many of these nurses' texts, as they apply their understanding of medical vision to their understanding of the war. What is on the surface? What is concealed? How does the nurse's examination intersect with the patient's own gaze? My analysis draws foremost on the writings of Ellen N. La Motte (1873–1961), whose radical innovations bear comparison to strategies in writings by various other nurses such as her coworker Mary Borden (1886–1968), who set up and funded l'Hôpital Chirurgical Mobile No. 1 in July 1915, within the French military system, staffed by French doctors and English-speaking nurses. La Motte dedicated her 1916 volume *The Backwash of War* "to Mary Borden-Turner 'The Little Boss' to whom I owe my experience in the zone of the armies." Yet Borden's dramatic use of the gaze discussed by Hazel Hutchison elsewhere in this volume often assumes "a high-wire aerial perspective" that "places the artist in a privileged" position, in contrast to the questioning and questing we find in La Motte, whose night nurse seeks to probe the hearts of her patients. Similar structures and concerns that complicate our notion of what we see are manifest in works by other nurses, from among whom I will draw samples by the Russian Lidiia Zakharova (born ca. 1888?), the Italian Maria Luisa Perduca (1896–1966), and the Romanian writer Hortensia Papadat-Bengescu (1876–1955), who worked on three very different military fronts.[16] These nurses' accounts address the difficulty of scientific observation, made evident by conflicts among medical observers. Moreover, the language of the nursing sister sometimes evokes the spiritual vigil by analogy to the healing vigil, watching over while also seeking illumination. Thus the multiplication of types of "looks" compounds and complicates our understanding of the task and the desires of the nurse.

My starting point is Ellen La Motte, a specialist in tuberculosis and opium addiction, who moved with her partner, Emily Chadbourne, in the gay circles of Chicago, London, Paris, and New York, and who visited Gertrude Stein's salon in Paris, where the importance of philosophers William James and Henri Bergson for thinking about painterly and literary cubism had been elaborated. For nearly two years from 1915 to 1916, La Motte worked in Paris at the American Hospital in Neuilly and then in Mary Borden's military "Hospital No. 1" as it moved along the front in Belgium and in northern France, before it was relocated in the Somme. Despite Claire Tylee's pathbreaking discussion in *The Great War and Women's Consciousness* (1990), La Motte's *Backwash of War* (1916), has received little attention, perhaps because her satiric, shifting narrative stance challenges the reader's attempts to interpret the conflicts and contradictions of wartime medicine. As the title *Backwash* suggests, La Motte's aim is to expose the dark side of war, showing the physical wreckage and the "dirty sediment at the bottom of most souls."[17] Her previous book on the treatment of tuberculosis and her subsequent work in China on the opium trade both stress the importance of environment and social control for health. It is not, therefore, surprising that she understands war injuries treated in a frontline hospital in Belgium as a political matter. She tackles the medical institutions of war in order to show hidden sides of war itself. Her vision can be compared not only to that of Mary Borden, her *Directrice*, whose body of prose appeared over ten years later, but also to that of other nurses such as the Frenchwoman Léonie Godfroy. As she began to write, Godfroy reflected, "I realized that the tableaux I was going to evoke differed in fundamental ways from most of those you see in the newspapers every day. This is caused by a difference in point of view. . . . War appears to be something abominable or something sublime, depending upon the side one experiences. I must declare that I saw only the somber side. This is women's share . . . the other side of the picture."[18] Cubist techniques expose aspects other than the heroic face of war; they make it possible to show not only the public, frontal side of medical practice in wartime, but also the back side that is normally concealed.

In her sketches, La Motte challenges traditional, idealizing views of war and bandaged visions of truth and justice by deploying several kinds of split perspective. In "Heroes" (1915), her first sketch, the night nurse carries a candle, like Diogenes the Cynic, searching for a true hero to compare to the man whose attempted suicide has brought him to her care. As a would-be suicide, he is considered by the military authorities as a deserter, who must be healed in order to be "stood up against a wall and shot." Tellingly, the revolver shot that brings the soldier to the operating room "tore out his left eye" (15). With his good eye, he fixes his gaze on *La Directrice*, then aims his "coward blood" (17) at her, staining her white uniform. The right eye becomes an instrument of his social rebellion, shooting blood onto those who would heal him—whether to execute him or to send him back to the killing fields. Thus from the first page of La Motte's book, the eye of the patient looks back. Surrounded by members of the medical staff who wait for the ether to take effect, he makes himself into a spectacle. His suicide attempt links him to shirkers, those whose self-inflicted wounds are simulacra of combat-wounds; such actions make them into distorting mirrors of war who comment on both their own character and the character of war.

La Motte's wry puns offer a verbal equivalent of the "double image." The nurse's task of healing a suicidal prisoner so that he can be court-martialed and executed, the narrator remarks, "seemed a dead-end occupation" (19, 22). This exceptional case highlights the underlying contradiction of military medicine, which subverts the Hippocratic oath "Do no harm," because it saves lives in order to enable further killing.[19] The narrator, who appears to be a day nurse, voices her distance from all the other characters—the unreasonable, hysterical, and "cowardly" suicide, the doctor coldly calculating the cost of ether, or the other medal-winning patients. Her perspective, however, like that of the doctor, is also largely economic. This day nurse may exemplify the splitting of personality described by Sandor Ferenczi that follows shock, where "emotions become severed from representations."[20] The night nurse, who takes her candle to watch over the men, observes them, "given to reflection" (20). By implication, she is a mirror who both reflects the pitiful wounded men and reflects on their selfishness, vanity, greed, and filthy jokes. Her candle goes out just as she realizes she can distinguish no difference between the suicide and the heroes. On taking another candle, however, "suddenly she saw" that the ideals for which the fighters sacrifice themselves are "compulsory" (23). Only one bloodied prisoner has refused that compulsion. The reader is left to ask whether his rebellion stands for a higher idealism that rejects patriotic militarism. To "see" in this sketch is to interpret and to judge. But blindness here is closely allied to insight, as Paul de Man argued.[21]

Just as a gunshot has given the nameless suicide of "Heroes" an "erratic eye" that has spilled out of place, a hemorrhage has given the protagonist Rochard of "Alone" "one blind, red eye that stared into Hell" (66)—straight ahead, unwinkingly—while his "dull, white eye" with the lid turned up shows his hold on life. In his split gaze, "it seemed as if the red, staring eye was looking for something the hospital could not give. And it seemed as if the white, glazed eye was indifferent to everything the hospital could give" (67–68). The nurse and the orderlies watch him and "regard" him, "but there was no one there to love him . . . to see beyond the horror" (67) of his two damaged eyes. The night nurse and the day nurse give him morphine and turn his body, but there is nothing further they can do, since Rochard has gas gangrene as well as a piece of shell lodged in his brain. Using a "beautiful expensive machine" donated by Madame Curie, the "radiographist"/anatomist has located the shrapnel, making the invisible visible, but he cannot operate. The soldier has become a "case" whom the students crowd round "to see" (60), a situation of observation in which these apprentices are passive, just as the medical staff are impotent. He has become a spectacle. These are students who receive merely two months' training at the field hospital, since "it was necessary to furbish up the immature and the senile" (60). They observe with their fingers, listening to the crackling bubbles symptomatic of "gas gangrene." They look at but cannot cure Rochard. Sight, in short, does not produce effective knowledge. Moreover, the medical staff produce agony in probing for knowledge by debridement of dead flesh and by applying carbolic acid that kills good tissue as well as germs. As the narrator explains, "the science of healing stood baffled before the science of destroying" (65). Both the narrator as a nurse and La Motte as a nurse-author indict the system that sacrifices "Little Rochard," a thirty-nine-year-old gardener, leaving to his child only his useless medal honoring "Valeur et Discipline." The beautiful machine contrasts ironically with the weak recruits that remain available for medical practice in wartime. What distinguishes La Motte's dark satire from many other nursing accounts, however, is the space she grants to the patient's return of the medical gaze, with two different eyes, neither of which retains conventional vision, but both of which speak through their gaze. The hospital has become a mirror site, in which the indifference of the staff meets Rochard's own stoic indifference to what the staff can give him, leaving him profoundly alone. La Motte here uses her bleak medical humor to examine the hypocrisies of the system that makes war and breaks men.

La Motte's splitting of the narrative voice may be most disturbing in her sketch "Women and Wives," a psychological study rather than a medical study. The very title thrusts into view the duplicity of official policies that distinguish wives (not permitted at the front, since they would lower morale) from "women," who may be local Belgian women or prostitutes of different qualities for soldiers of different ranks, who "cheer and refresh the troops" (111). The narrator cannot explain the rule. "It is rather paradoxical, but there are those who can explain it perfectly" (111). The opening description of "ordinary" bitter winter weather sets a naturalist stage for the conversation among the patients around the stove in which worn photographs of working-class wives symbolize the demographics of wartime sacrifice. Home, with what she calls the "little, ugly . . . stupid, ordinary wives" appears for the moment at least to be of more interest to these men than "the glories and heroisms of war" (107). Yet the narrator complains that each of these men regularly visits a local woman—even a little girl of fourteen in the village. As the narrator moves from the photographs to the wives, then to the kept "women," she pauses twice to note: "I don't understand" (111, 113). Her task, however, is to record the contradiction. "I must write you of what I have seen, the other side, the backwash. They are both true" (112). The contradictory attitudes of her male colleagues toward their families and toward their sexual partners require a multifaceted representation in which the narrator herself cannot retain a single perch from which to judge these men.

The narrator then turns to challenge the reader: "Have you ever watched . . . Have you seen the girls . . . ?" (114). We might compare Mary Borden's "Belgium", the first story in *The Forbidden Zone*, where the narrator insists on her factual control in dialogue with the reader: "Come, I'll show you" (4).[22] The only explanation La Motte's narrator offers for these bothersome discontinuities must be that the Belgian girls on the Allied side are guilty of seducing the decent soldiers, of spying, while the Germans on the occupied side are "brutes" who force women to sleep with them. As the narrator proposes this patriotic explanation, assigning responsibility to women on one side but to the men on the other, she exclaims to us, "Can't you see? You must be pro-German!" (115). Here the play of perspective confronts the reader with the narrator's ugly, contradictory angle of vision that may or may not coincide with the darkly pessimistic quotations of official judgments that pepper the narrator's descriptions. La Motte deploys strategies of realism—detailed descriptions, well-fingered photographs, and unreliable narrator—to underscore the ordinariness of sexual drives and the hypocrisy of the rules that govern the militarized zone (which Mary Borden calls "the forbidden zone"), as well as the implausibility of the distinctions between ally and enemy. The men she mocks come from every rank: the orderlies, the young surgeon, the hospital purveyor, and the sixty-four-year-old doctor, or *Médecin chef*. Beyond their self-contradictions, she sees the corrosive effects of the system on the women themselves. As readers, whom she is inviting to "see" this reality, we are particularly disoriented by the conventionally patriotic language that the narrator uses to defend the men. For example, she couples exaggeration with understatement. "War, superb as it is, is not necessarily a filtering process" (112). To see, to observe, to watch becomes difficult for us, when she slides from her disabused exposition to her patriotic critiques of Germans (and of the women who are their putative victims), zigzagging from one irony to the next. The contradictory positioning of the narrator in this way destabilizes the belligerent nationalism that governs military policy in the frontline zone, under whose regime the mobile hospital falls, inviting the reader to rethink the multiple binaries that govern this zone—between us and them, between superior officers and peasants, and between "women" and "wives." The "double image" as a structural principle of displacement is perfectly exemplified by the narrator's comment that there is both a heroic side and the "other" side of war, "the backwash. They are both true" (112). Equally important, however, is the interpellation of the reader, who is called on to "see" the social landscape, in the sense of explicate; the reader must interrogate the picture of the hospital that the narrator presents, with all its moral obfuscations and gendered contradictions. When La Motte's narrator writes, "I must write you of what I have seen," she presses us, her readers, to "see" the same; however, the contradictory behaviors she records are too puzzling to permit clear moral understanding. "There are those who can explain it perfectly"—but not the narrator, who realizes that "everything has two sides" (111). La Motte's focus on the "Backwash" makes her sketches much gloomier than many other nursing texts, with the possible exception of those by Borden and Madeleine Clemenceau-Jacquemaire. That this critique of patriotism, of hypocrisy, of incompetence appeared in 1916 is astonishing; it was possible only in a neutral state, before the US declared war in 1917. Even in retrospect, La Motte's texts stand out by their experimental complexity of narrative structure.

La Motte's sketches in *The Backwash of War* are closely related to those written by her *Directrice* Mary Borden over the four years of her hospital work and published a decade after the war in 1929. As a number of critics, including Carol Acton, Santanu Das, Jane Marcus, and Claire Tylee, have noted, many of Borden's disabused sketches and stories also direct a searchlight onto the themes of blindness and insight, X-rays, and the medical need to apply multiple senses, like multiple angles, to the healing of patients.[23] One brief satire, "Sentinels," for example, calls our attention to the futility of visual inspection, when the guard who reads the papers of each passerby has no way to verify a name or identity. Rather than discover a distinct mission or person, the sentinel's inspection "is always the same": it locates nothing specific to this moment and this encounter.[24] Instead of a multiplication of perspectives on "the generals who do not look and the colonels who glance sideways" (21), there is a collapse of multiple viewings into one. "Viser," that is, to view in the sense of certify or inspect, is impossible. As another sketch indicates, men are deformed by war, all "in the same way." "The same machine had twisted and bent them all" (27). Borden intensifies this sameness by a rhetoric of repetition and negation, underscoring what the men (and we) do not know as well as what they do know. Other sketches take up and challenge the "plurisensorial" methods that Foucault writes about. Thus "Paraphernalia" interpellates the nurse whose accumulated "things" (bottles, tubes, liquids, saws, and syringes) will be defeated by "inexorable" death. No effort at interpretation or intervention, no sensory perception (whether sight or hearing) can avail to heal. In an age when "the X-ray photograph was . . . viewed by some spiritualists as an image of the soul,"[25] Borden steers between the two. "The man's spirit is invisible. Why do you light the lamp?

You cannot see the God of Death with your splendid eyes" (132). Borden was certainly not a believer in the spiritualism that, as Jay Winter explains, gave comfort to grieving survivors of the war.[26] Indeed, part of the power of "Enfant de Malheur," about the death of a Parisian "apache" or criminal, springs from Borden's juxtaposition of different ideological responses to death: the terrified sewer rat who looks like a Greek god, the frigid Madonna-like Protestant nurse Pim, the orderly Guerin, who is also a dedicated Catholic priest, and the nurse-narrator, who rejects supernatural beliefs, saying to herself that "soon he'll be nothing, nothing" (88). Although to each a different "child of sorrow" appears, it is Guerin who will bring the relief of forgiveness to the violent soldier, who becomes a "boy" again at the end (91–92). Unlike La Motte, Borden in her sketches may follow up the fracturing of her picture with a positive resolution into coherence that emphasizes understanding and mutual support.

Borden's preface describes her sketches as "fragments of a great confusion" that cannot be reduced to "order." Her fragmented perspective, allied to the cubist strategies of La Motte, is undoubtedly most conspicuous in a semi-dramatic sketch spoken in several anonymous voices, "In the Operating Room" (134–43). Laid out as a play with bits of bridging narrative, this sketch records the cacophony of an operating room, where three surgeons and their three patients, nameless nurses, and an officer exchange snippets of conversation, which underscore the hopelessness of most operations. By assimilating military surgery to the assembly line of industrial production, in which nameless men undergo triage by body part and medical specialty (abdomen, lung, knee), she exposes the disassembly of the body and of the human being in wartime. Ricocheting pleas and comments frame the 3rd Patient's dying observation: "I cannot see. I cannot see any more . . . It is dark." Spliced between this patient's despairing words about his dying loss of sight are the 3rd Surgeon's technical assessments on cutting open the bandage: "I can do nothing . . . Too late" (141). A death has been silently buried here, as the conversation moves on. If a cubist painting breaks up the body along different planes in space, this cubist play gives voice to patient and surgeon without any real interchange. Rather than connect these two partners in the operation, the play disconnects the doctors from their frantic work, focusing ironically on the pleasure of oysters to come. Borden fragments the diagnostic dialogues to shatter our sense of organic healing.

In her two best-known stories, "Moonlight" and "Blind," vision collaborates with the other senses, as the narrator listens to the sounds of war and pain or senses the odors of the harvest and the medications. The moonlight in the first story doubles itself by reflections in a pail or in a pool of water on the floor, yet sets itself off as a romantic image from the actual world of death and wounds. Like the moon, the narrator doubles herself as a second nurse carrying a lantern into the gangrene ward, a woman who can survive only by killing her own heart, deafening herself, and blinding herself: "Blind, deaf, dead" (64). The many patients' eyes ("eyes of sick dogs, sick cats, blind eyes, eyes of delirium"), set into "torn parts" of men, echo in their blindness her own self-imposed anesthesia, as Jane Marcus has pointed out, which blunts her ability to observe. The moment of recognition, when she understands that she cannot continue living when faced with the destruction of the men all about her, comes as a patient looks back and retains his humanity: "a man looks up at me from the shambles"—signaling, smiling even, with a heroism that "blinds" her with its brilliance (64). Indirectly, the metaphor of the moon implies the sun of technological knowledge that shines and illuminates the medical work performed in the hospital. This moonlight is saturated with the perfume of harvest, emblem of romance; the image is complicated, because the harvest is trope for the dead, and the odor of the hay fuses with the stench of gangrene. While Borden's poetry links her own face to the moon as a reflection of her erotic response to her lover, here the theme of romance is dismissed as dangerous, a form of blind sentimentality that can only distract from the battle for life taking place within the hospital. Yet the blinding gaze of the soldier connects the symbolism of the sun to the uncomplaining stoicism and heroism of those who are dying, returning us to what we may deem traditional values.

Blindness takes similarly paradoxical forms in the companion story "Blind" that Borden wrote in the late 1920s. The nurse-narrator sees stretcher-bearers, who look for space in a crowded wooden "baraque" (hut) to bring in a bandaged soldier, who takes the place of a dead "boy" she has been holding in her arms, like a Pietà. Borden captures the dreamlike confusion of the ward, subdivided by wooden screens that conceal the dressing area and kitchen, and the narrator explains that she watches the new patient "out of the corner of my eye," while working with a brilliant surgeon (147). She scans the carpet of men "for my special secret signals" (163). Her "acute eyes" watch for the scurrying "unseen thing"—Death (160). She knows the new patient is blind, because it is written on his ticket, but he does not yet know this. His blindness is not knowledge or power here; it points to the impossible exchange of gaze between the nurse and the soldier, whom she had forgotten. The nurse does triage under pressure, using not only her long-distance observation of twitches or color, but also her touch, as Das has pointed out.[27] The surgeons with "feverish" eyes wield their knives against "the invisible enemy" death. The narrator looks back at herself in the past, as one might look at a mirror. What she "sees" through a mist is "some strange dream-hell where I am glad to be employed" (155), bound together with the injured and the orderlies. Dramatically playing with a syntactic shift, Borden offers us here a split gaze at her own incomprehensible self in the past—"that woman, myself"—at the edge of succumbing to the strains of her work (160). Whereas the cubist project orients its epistemological investigation in space, Borden in 1929 orients her metanarrative comments across time, testing the meaning of her work in relationship to the intense state of semiconsciousness that shaped her knowledge of war but that memory suggests may have been a "dream."

One of the most striking examples of the problematic motif of the "invisible visible" in wartime nursing narratives appears in the novel *Balaurul* (The Dragon, 1923) by Hortensia Papadat-Bengescu.[28] A symbolist Romanian writer, Papadat-Bengescu served in 1918 as a Red Cross nurse at Focsani, where her husband was assigned to serve. In the tenth chapter of that book, entitled "The Man Whose Heart They Could See," Papadat-Bengescu traces the encounter of Laura, a naive and idealistic nurse assigned to provide ambulatory care at a train station, with a hospitalized casualty whose wound had been scraped by a shell that removed the surface of his chest, exposing his beating heart. He has become a spectacle for all the personnel to come observe: "Have you seen? You have to see! . . . Such horror!" (357). W. J. T. Mitchell notes, "we live in a culture of images, a society of the spectacle,"[29] and Papadat-Bengescu, like Mary Borden, depicts the medical ward as a theater, where the doctor commands his assistant, "Look!" (359). Surprisingly, this hypervisual context frames an impossibility of seeing or even imagining. From the outset the gentle narrator considers all the ways in which the "naked soul" can be revealed—through the eyes, the lips, the honest word, the hand that allow us to see a person's "mysterious heart" (356). In the backdrop of her reflections we learn of the misery to which she has been exposed, whether by the mismanagement of the hospital that left incompetent internists to perform surgery as "endless hacking," or by the ingenuity of wounds that break skulls, grind flesh, and "blindly" destroy. Such blind surgery is indifferent to the consequences of its action. These evocations prepare us for what she will discover and its larger metaphorical scope.

As Laura approaches the soldier's bed, she imagines the intact organ (an "altar" unveiled) beating and shuts in her feelings apprehensively. But when she reaches him, she cannot see—she can only hear a "strange and disquieting whistling noise." The object of Laura's gaze, a strong, blond, and handsome peasant, whom she admires at first glance, is also the topic of rumors, gossip, the babble of staff at the station infirmary and the hospital that obscure his identity as "the Man." The Man himself is afraid to see his own body, and her own glance is so swift that she does not perhaps ever see his heart. To "see" the heart would mean to see the suffering of the man, who attempts to tear off the bandages that hurt him and who tries to scratch the itching wound that has become his new "enemy" (361). He has become a "martyr," an echo of Christ and an "effigy of pain"—that is, a simulacrum of the pain that cannot otherwise be shown. With his hands bound to prevent him from lacerating himself, he calls on Laura to "see how they tie me!" She must "see" and bear witness to his confinement not only by his wound, but also by an institution that performs futile rituals of healing. For six days, this conflict between life and death besieges the "primitive icon" of a lacerated chest. Laura continues to work in the intensive care unit, then checks on him, becoming "a poor priestess of hopeless pain" for whom observation and minimal comforts have displaced healing. She keeps vigil as the patients sleep or turn in torment. Crammed into a corridor with others who are dying, the Man now quarrels with a second soldier, whose mouth has been devoured by worms. Each disgusted by the other, "they lay there glued to each other; one with his glazed blue eyes fixed on the wormy mouth; the other fascinated by the hideous opening inside which the heart was choking" (362). The narrator lines up the two indignant patients' exchange of horrified gazes, whose "glazed" fixation interrupts comprehension, and contrasts them to Laura's unremitting yet serene effort to find and soothe them. The relay of gazes creates a dizzying hall of mirrors in which each grotesque manifestation of the war compounds the next. Meanwhile, the doctor simply comments that this "had been indeed a unique case in the museum of war surgery" (362). Jon Dietrick argues, "In a powerful critique of [the] conception of visual perception as an unmediated, objective and passive process for the viewer, Papadat-Bengescu demonstrates, via Laura's failure to see, that the imaginary constructions we erect necessarily set limits to what we can 'see.'"[30] As Dietrick elucidates, Papadat-Bengescu "complicates the relationship between 'seeing' and 'knowing.'"[31]

In this chapter of her war-novel, Papadat-Bengescu offers a complex revision of the usual surface/depth distinction implied in Foucault's "invisible visibility." While the "sacred organ" of the heart may be visible, its inaccessibility to Laura underscores her idealizing projection onto the body of a soldier whose self-destructive acts and rage at those around him betray his "heart" in another sense. Over the course of the chapter, Laura comes to grasp the "new and strange epidemics" and gangrenes that spring from the international spread of innovative means of destruction, introducing new "flora specific to modern wars," flora that feed "the vampire of war." Paradoxically, destructive technological innovations are naturalized as flora that the scientist can observe. For Laura, however, the medical observation becomes an allegory for a social critique and a gaze at the moral pathology of war. As she leads us up to the deaths of the two juxtaposed men, she uses death itself as what Foucault calls "the absolute point of view over life and opening . . . on its truth."[32]

The averted gaze of the witness who cannot bear to see is a motif that Papadat-Bengescu shares with many other nurse-observers. If Laura "sees" the exposed heart only by looking at the eyes of the doctor, in a triangulated perspective, other nurses avert their gaze in a struggle to endorse one truth rather than another. As Borden writes of the nurse who anesthetizes herself, "she is blind so that she cannot see the torn parts of men she must handle" (64). Or in Maria Luisa Perduca's story, "An Amputation" (1915), when an Italian amputee woke up without memory of his lost leg and "looked at us and smiled," the novice nurse-narrator reports, "We had to look the other way to hide our faces."[33] Paradoxically, the patient's knowledge or repression of knowledge may be as powerful an agent of truth as the nurse's and may offer an equally potent social commentary.

While variations on the theme of sight—the gaze, the examination, the spectacle—are commonly situated in the theater of the operating room or the hospital, those nurses who were serving on a mobile front might be sent onto the battlefield itself to pick up the injured. This violation of old gender norms that allow men to "see" battle but keep women behind the lines may explain why the theme acquires peculiar power in that context. A rich chapter in Lidiia Zakharova's *Dnevnik Sestry Miloserdiia na peredovykh positiiakh* (Diary of a Red Cross Sister in the Front Lines, 1915) recounts her first encounter with an actual battlefield, passing from a seized enemy trench into No Man's Land, then back to her own comrades. Her vivid description of the landscape at dusk captures the problematic nature of the gaze, which cannot distinguish the living from the dead, nor the Russian from the German wounded. The trenches are a complex labyrinth of corridors and "blind alleys" that challenge anyone who tries to pass through. They are filled with furnishings (displacing the "home" into the trench) and other valuables collected by the German soldiers—like a scrapbook devoted to the war, to be read by those who follow. In a dugout, not a person but a toppled child's high chair is a "mute witness" to the bloody drama. As an inscribed viewer, the chair without its child "made even more horrifying and monstrous the sight of trenches overflowing with masses of dead bodies." Zakharova describes this "gruesome spectacle" as if it were a frozen pantomime, its actors in "poses that made them seem alive."[34] What the nurse finds most terrible is the sight of soldiers still standing, leaning on the parapet, "eyes open and glazed with the tranquility of non-existence" (185). In this topsy-turvy world it is difficult to know who is the witness, which the knower and which the known. While the orderlies head back to the field station, Zakharova continues to hunt for her wounded, and she becomes disoriented. To "look" is to seek, but she is led inadvertently to the enemy, who amicably exchange prisoners and thereby overturn the categories of desire and fear within which she has operated. The proximity of the two sides finds an ironic echo later, when she has delivered the wounded and sick to a market town, where everyday business streams by, only a few *versts* (kilometers) from the "bloody tragedy of war": "the quiet, provincial life I was observing was streaming along a crater more treacherous and uncertain than the crater of a volcano" (186). While she has passed in her cart from one world to the other, observing both, the inhabitants of the "mundane" world are as blind as the dead soldiers whose eyes remain open. To observe the meaning of war requires that she also attempt to observe the meaning of peace.

Each of these writers' explorations of the nurse's medical gaze builds up tensions that strain meaning. Realism conflicts with destabilizing devices. These writers observe grotesque details such as the sparkling blood on the nails of Laura's patient, after he has torn at his wound, in Papadat-Bengescu's "The Man," or the suicide's "two big teeth" broken by the mouth gag imposed to keep him quiet while the doctor trephines his skull in La Motte's story "Heroes." While La Motte records the moral judgments and medical bookkeeping of the doctor who works on this patient in "Heroes," she also splits open the moral dilemmas of wartime nursing by splitting her own narrative voice into a dialogue of self-interrogation and contradiction. Furthermore, the unstable connotations of the vocabulary—the "erratic" eye that the doctor binds back in place—release those details from the function of the real to provoke larger questions about medical and social dysfunctions. A familiar distinction between a nurse and a doctor recurs in these scenes—the nurse exploring the moral meaning of her task while the doctor calmly performs a cost-benefit analysis and perceives the suffering human victim as a scientific "case" to be classified in a "museum of war surgery" (Papadat-Bengescu, "The Man," 362). Yet distinctions between figures are also blurred, as one mimics or ventriloquizes the voice of another. The evolution of the patient's condition appears like a stroboscopic sequence of snapshots in which a form that first appears soon takes on quite another shape and larger meaning. Invisibly at first, then perceptibly, the wound opens up and unfolds the structures within which it is framed. In wartime sketches of patients, narrative lays out as a temporal sequence what painting might lay out in space, as we observe the progressive evolution of the suicide, of "Little Rochard," or of "the Man" whose heart you could see.

Through their ironic juxtapositions and multiplied angles of vision, these nurse-writers exemplify Mikhail Bakhtin's observation about humor's "remarkable power of making an object come up close, of drawing it into a zone of crude contact where one can finger it familiarly on all sides, turn it upside down, inside out, peer at it from above and below . . . look into its center, doubt it, take it apart, dismember it, lay it bare and expose it."[35] Most dramatically, some of these writers, from La Motte to Papadat-Bengescu, wrench the gaze away from the doctor or the *Directrice* and give space to the patient's own gaze, thereby reversing the relationship of power that for Foucault resided in the panopticon. The nameless giant in "Heroes" who eyes the *Directrice*, poor Rochard with his white and his red eyes, or the blinding smile of Borden's brave patient all become endowed with an agency of the eye to which the narrator and the reader must respond. Even the immobile dead in Zakharova's uncanny landscape of death have open eyes: they, too, bear mute witness in a war that has become a trial of mankind's humanity.

In *A Room of One's Own* (1929), Virginia Woolf proposes that we "turn history wrong side out" to expose its underside.[36] She describes a "sudden splitting of consciousness . . . when from being the natural inheritor" of a civilization, a woman "becomes on the contrary, outside of it, alien and critical."[37] Woolf's proposal perfectly fits that project of Ellen La Motte and of other nurses during the Great War. To turn the history of war "wrong side out," these women artists and writers were forced to split their consciousness of what they saw. In different ways, that self-division could serve to test the evidence, like the double-blind experiments of Dr. Rivers. And to do this, they were able to draw on the tools that cubism offered, to expose the hidden sides of the war, as well as on the new medical technologies like the X-ray that had been made available to them to represent the impact of the war. Testimony thus becomes a test of integrity, an inquiry into the truths of war as well as into the changed nature of the self of the writer.

NOTES

1. V. Brittain, *Verses of a V.A.D.*, foreword by M. C. Leighton (London: E. Macdonald, 1918).
2. M. Foucault, *The Birth of the Clinic: An Archaeology of Medical Perception*, trans. A. M. Sheridan Smith (New York: Pantheon, 1973 [1963]).
3. A. Becker, "The Avant-Garde, Madness and the Great War," *Journal of Contemporary History* 35, no. 1 (2000): 76.
4. S. Das, *Touch and Intimacy in First World War Literature* (Cambridge: Cambridge University Press, 2005).
5. M. Curie, *La Radiologie et la guerre* (Paris: Fayard, 1921), 71, 77.
6. Foucault, *The Birth*, 165–66.
7. M. Higonnet, "X-Ray Vision: Women Photograph War," *Miranda* 2 (July 2010). Available online at http://www.miranda-ejournal.eu/1/miranda/article.xsp?numero=2&id_article=article_22-548.
8. C. M. Tylee, "The Spectacle of War: Photographs of the Russian Front by Florence Farmborough," *Women: A Cultural Review* 8, no. 1 (1997): 65–80.
9. J. Marcus, "Afterword," in *Not So Quiet . . .* (New York: Feminist Press, 1989), 268; Tylee, *The Great War.*
10. J. Gallagher, *The World Wars through the Female Gaze* (Carbondale: Southern Illinois University Press, 1998), 6.
11. E. J. Leed, *No Man's Land: Combat and Identity in World War I* (New York: Cambridge University Press, 1979), 124.
12. D. Cottington, *Cubism in the Shadow of War: The Avant-Garde and Politics in Paris 1905–1914* (New Haven, CT: Yale University Press, 1988), 123.
13. P. Leighten, "Picasso's Collages and the Threat of War, 1912–13," *Art Bulletin* 67, no. 4 (1985): 653; P. Leighten, *Re-Ordering the Universe: Picasso and Anarchism, 1897–1914* (Princeton, NJ: Princeton University Press, 1989).
14. M. Antliff and P. Leighten, *Cubism and Culture* (New York: Thames and Hudson, 2001), chap. 2, 6.
15. Leed, *No Man's Land*, 137.
16. Beyond what she wrote in her memoir, *Dnevnik Sestry Miloserdiia na peredovykh positiiakh* (St. Petersburg: Izdatel'stvo Biblioteka "Velikoi Voiny," 1915), we know little about Zakharova, a middle-class Russian mother who left her children with their grandmother in order to follow her husband to the front, but was forced by illness to return home after several months; she may have had an affair with cavalry officer Georgy Zhukov. Maria Luisa Perduca, a young French teacher, won numerous medals for her medical service during the two World Wars. Hortensia Papadat-Bengescu was an admired member of the Romanian avant-garde, who served as a Red Cross nurse in Focsani during the war and recorded the minutiae of her observations in what she called a "document-novel."
17. La Motte, *Backwash*, 112. Further references are included parenthetically in the text.
18. L. Godfroy, *Souvenirs d'ambulance et de captivité (Noyon à Holzminden)* (Paris: L'Eclair, 1917), 5.
19. Publishing in 1919, Madeleine Clemenceau-Jacquemaire, daughter of the prime minister, likewise condemned the moral contradictions of military medicine that patches men up only to torture their bodies another time, with

the turn of the wheel that brings them back wounded five or six times; see "Rentrants," *L'Illustration* 3969 (29 March 1919): 353.

20. S. Ferenczi, "Trauma and Splitting of the Personality," in *The Clinical Diary of Sandor Ferenczi*, ed. J. Dupont, trans. M. Balint and N. Zarday Jackson (Cambridge, MA: Harvard University Press, 1988 [1932]), 203.
21. P. de Man, *Blindness and Insight: Essays in the Rhetoric of Contemporary Criticism*, 2nd ed., introduction by W. Godzich (London: Methuen, 1983).
22. In "Belgium", the first story in *The Forbidden Zone*, Mary Borden insists on her factual control in dialogue with the reader: "Come, I'll show you" (4), in *The Forbidden Zone* (Garden City, NY: Doubleday, Doran, 1930). See Hazel Hutchison's extensive discussion of vision in Borden's work in this volume.
23. C. Acton, *Grief in Wartime: Private Pain, Public Discourse* (Basingstoke: Palgrave MacMillan, 2007).
24. Borden, *Forbidden Zone*, 18. Further references are included parenthetically in the text.
25. L. Cartwright, *Screening the Body: Tracing Medicine's Visual Culture* (Minneapolis: University of Minnesota Press, 1995), 121.
26. J. Winter, *Sites of Memory, Sites of Mourning: The Great War in European Cultural History* (Cambridge: Cambridge University Press, 1995), 54–77.
27. H. Hutchison locates the power of life or death in the hands of the nurse narrator as "fate."
28. H. Papadat-Bengescu, "The Man Whose Heart You Could See," trans. D. Stetco, in M. Higonnet, *Lines of Fire: Women Writers of World War I* (New York: Penguin Plume, 1999), 356–62. Further references are included parenthetically in the text.
29. W. J. T. Mitchell, *Picture Theory* (Chicago: Chicago University Press, 1994), 5.
30. J. Dietrick, "Seeing Battle, Knowing War: Feminist Re-Visioning in Hortensia Papadat-Bengescu's 'The Man Whose Heart They Could See,'" *Journal of International Women's Studies* 4, no. 3 (2003): 103.
31. Ibid., 102.
32. Foucault, *The Birth*, 155.
33. M. L. Perduca, "An Amputation," trans. S. Notini, in M. Higonnet, *Lines of Fire: Women Writers of World War I* (New York: Penguin Plume, 1999), 219.
34. L. Zakharova, "Diary of a Red-Cross Sister in the Front Lines," trans. C. Simmons, in M. Higonnet, *Lines of Fire: Women Writers of World War I* (New York: Penguin Plume, 1999), 185. Further references are included parenthetically in the text.
35. M. Bakhtin, *The Dialogic Imagination. Four Essays*, trans. C. Emerson and M. Holquist (Austin: University of Texas Press, 1981), 23.
36. V. Woolf, *A Room of One's Own* (New York: Harcourt Brace, 1929), 44.
37. Ibid., 93.

Afterword

Remembering the First World War Nurse in Britain and France

Alison S. Fell

After the Armistice, the figure that was set up most frequently as the female equivalent to the combatant male in discourses of commemoration in all of the belligerent nations was that of the middle- or upper-class volunteer nurse, whose activities could be most straightforwardly mapped onto the well-established model of nineteenth-century charitable work among elite women, and who did not present any competition to demobilized men in the employment market.[1] The contribution of trained nurses was also generally positively represented postwar, although their war service was not always praised as highly or as frequently as that of untrained nurses, something that irked many professional and military nurses. A 1919 letter published in *The Times*, for example, demanded to know why "a regular Matron of the official Army Nursing Service, who has served throughout the war, may lay no claim to the war medal which is awarded to any VAD . . . not technically in the army at all, with possibly only a few weeks of service to her credit, during which she may have done little or no actual nursing."[2] That said, in terms of general postwar attitudes toward women's war work, in both Britain and France the nurse remained the most acceptable model of patriotic female war service.

In this chapter I examine, firstly, the function of the First World War nurse in national cultures of remembrance, and, secondly, the ways in which nurses themselves remembered their war work and the service and deaths of their colleagues. I argue that while the nurse tended to be cast in both British and French memorials and ceremonies to the war dead as the embodiment of abstract national values, or as an icon of patriotic femininity, nursing organizations themselves were keen to emphasize the risk to life and health of wartime nursing work, overtly drawing parallels with the war service and sacrifices of mobilized men. In a third section, I consider the representation of First World War nursing in more recent popular memories of the conflict, suggesting that just as in the interwar period, the temporary volunteer nurse has maintained a higher profile than the professional or military nurse. However, the dominant vision of nurses as self-abnegating, patriotic, and maternal was overlaid from the 1970s onward with a conceptualization of wartime nursing as an empowering enterprise for women that had liberated them from a prewar life of sheltered domesticity, a view of women's relationship to war that was influenced by second-wave feminist thinking. I conclude that both of these myths inevitably mask the diversity of experiences of French and British women who were engaged in wartime nursing work.

NATIONS REMEMBERING NURSES

The most common female figure in First World War memorials and ceremonies during the interwar years was the grieving woman, a figure that not only translated the mourning experienced by hundreds of thousands of widows and bereaved mothers, but that also functioned as the incarnation of a community's or a nation's grief.[3] However, women also appeared in other guises, and the nurse was the most popular cipher for female service and sacrifice both during the war and in the 1920s. The First World War nurse was set up as an idealized role model that had broad appeal, being easily subsumed into dominant conceptions of femininity while at the same time being positioned as a female equivalent of mass male mobilization. Many evocations of the wartime nurse thus drew on traditional understandings of women's rights and roles and offered reassuringly domesticated versions of mobilized women on active service during the war.[4] Yet while some memorials drew on conceptions of nursing as an extension of women's maternal and domestic role in order to make their wartime service embody abstract values such as humanity, civilization, reconciliation, and healing, others positioned nurses as citizens, their work being understood in this context as an admirable example of an individual's fulfillment of civic or patriotic duty to the nation.

Certain evocations of the nurse in the interwar years effectively combine the roles of nurse and grieving woman, with the nurse depicted as a Pietà with a dead or wounded soldier presented as a Christ figure. This is particularly the case in France, where interwar commemoration was permeated, as Annette Becker notes, by the "religious and mystical realm . . . when Judeo-Christian catechisms were entwined with the secular gospels of patriotism."[5] The war memorial in Charlieu (Loire) (Figure A.1) is of this type. Sculpted by Christian-Henri Roullier-Levasseur and unveiled in 1922, it features a nurse wearing a First World War uniform and cradling a dead French soldier, his helmet by his side. This rare appearance of a realist sculpture of a uniformed nurse on a French memorial is perhaps explained by the fact that the mayor of Charlieu was Dr. Jean-Louis Vitaud, who had worked as a doctor in the French army during the war.[6] A similar depiction of a nurse caring for a dying soldier can be found on a plaque in the Saint-Louis des Invalides chapel in Paris that is dedicated to French Red Cross nurses. In the foreground, a uniformed nurse is bandaging the wounds of a prostrate soldier, while in the background a ruined French village burns. Despite their contemporary dress, the nurses in these memorials are recognizable as Marian figures, as the ancient *Stabat Mater dolorosa*.

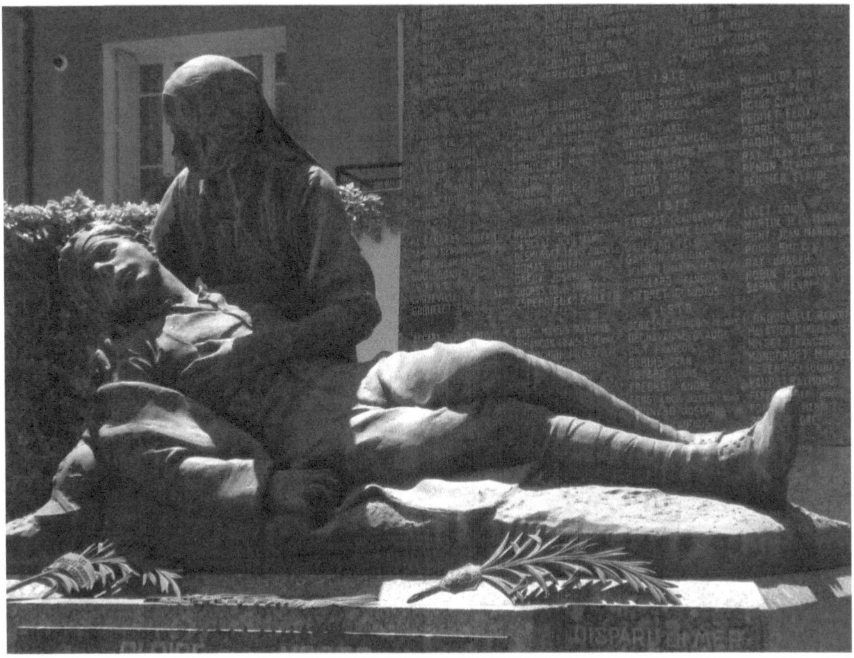

Figure A.1 War memorial, 1922, sculpted by Christian-Henri Roullier-Levasseur, Charlieu (Loire). Photograph courtesy of Marc Lacelle.

In Britain, however, nurses who appear on First World War memorials tend to be positioned in similar poses to soldiers, rather than in maternal, nurturing, or grieving mode. In this way, they serve to embody the sacrifices and contributions made by women to the war effort, a feminized version of masculine war service. Some of these memorials overtly position them as citizens, having "done their bit," despite the fact that there are very few women named on the list of the fallen. The war memorial in Bold Venture Park, Darwen, Lancashire, for example, sculpted by Louis Roslyn, features a tall square pedestal with bronze reliefs on three of its sides representing a soldier, a sailor, and a nurse, while at the top of the pedestal stands a winged figure representing Victory (Figure A.2).[7] The nurse here is also in First World War uniform, but unlike the French examples she is not evocative of religious iconography. Her sleeves are rolled up, she is carrying the tools of her trade like the soldier carries his rifle, and she wears a medal as proof of the value of her service to the state. Her dress, pose, and gaze mirror those of the war-weary men on the other reliefs. The memorial was unveiled on 27 September 1921. It is possible that Roslyn was influenced by George Frampton's 1920 memorial to Edith Cavell, as the word "Humanity" is engraved below the nurse, expressing a specifically female brand of wartime sacrifice, whereas beneath the male military figure is the word "Freedom."

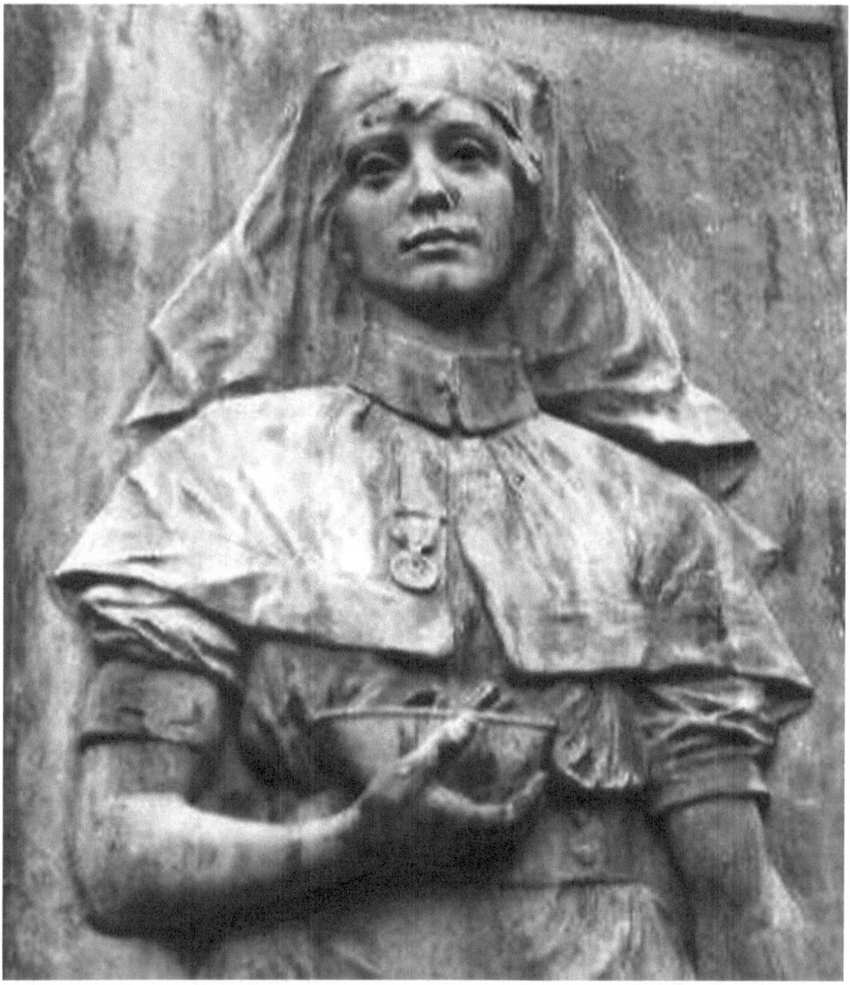

Figure A.2 War memorial, 1921, sculpted by Louis Roslyn, Bold Venture Park, Darwen, Lancashire. Photograph courtesy of Gordon T. Lawson.

In fact, the figure of Edith Cavell can be seen as a kind of "Urtext" behind many interwar representations of nursing, with what was perceived as her martyrdom functioning in the cultures of commemoration in both nations as the ultimate iconic version of patriotic self-abnegation. In interwar cultural representations produced in France and Britain, Cavell was made to embody two central (and frequently interlinked) concepts: the brutality of the enemy and the humanity and self-sacrifice of womanhood. These were concepts that many different sections of the national and international community could buy into. The former—that of an innocent nurse mercilessly gunned down by brutal Germans—dominated commemoration during the war and was instrumentalized by anti-German and, in Britain and the US, recruitment propagandists. They reimagined Cavell, a forty-nine-year-old professional nurse who had pleaded guilty to her role in organizing an escape network for Allied soldiers, as a young, virginal, and feeble war victim of a brutal oppressor that needed avenging, acting as a proxy for other vulnerable female civilians.[8]

The use of Cavell as a means of condemning the enemy was evident in the 1920 Paris memorial to Cavell sculpted by Gabriel Pech for the Jardin des Tuileries. Initiated by the newspaper *Le Matin*, which launched a competition for a Cavell memorial in 1916, and with a committee dominated by male republican politicians, the invitation to submit proposals sent to various French artists was clear about the messages the memorial was to convey: "By means of the pure and tender effigy of the English nurse, isn't it humanity itself, a victim of barbarism and demanding revenge, that deserves to be glorified?"[9] In Pech's winning interpretation, Cavell is depicted after her execution, prostrate among war-torn ruins while a German helmet symbolizing the brutality of the enemy lies on top of her body. Placed squarely within the Catholic framework of martyrdom, a female allegorical figure floats above her, holding a martyr's palm in one hand and scattering flowers on the victim with the other. Cavell's martyrdom was underlined in the unveiling ceremony, with André Maginot, the French Minister of Pensions, comparing Cavell, "the nurse-martyr," to Joan of Arc in his speech.[10] Its location, which was chosen unanimously by the committee, connotes Cavell's perceived importance via its prestige, and is given additional resonance by its proximity to James Pradier's statue of Strasbourg in the place de la Concorde, the symbol *par excellence* of anti-German sentiment in nineteenth-century France. The *revanchisme* evident in the French Cavell memorial helps to explain why it was destroyed by Nazi soldiers on their entry into Paris in 1940.[11]

The 1920 British memorial to Cavell, sculpted by George Frampton and situated in St Martin's Place in central London, has a similar genesis to its Parisian equivalent. It was also funded by public subscription initiated in the immediate aftermath of her death by a newspaper, the *Daily Telegraph*, and was unveiled on 17 March 1920. However, Frampton's interpretation depicts her at the moment of her execution and presents her as an older, dignified, and serene figure, bravely facing her executors and gazing toward the horizon. In her analysis, art historian Sue Malvern comments that the bearing and clothing of the Cavell figure "repress the signs of femininity," and Katie Pickles agrees that in some senses Cavell is represented as an "honorary man."[12] It is true that she is seen as dying for, rather than representing, innocent female victims (the vulnerable mother and child that top the monument are generally assumed to represent Belgium and Serbia). But Frampton draws above all on the tradition of the martyr-heroine, a tradition in which a particular brand of femininity—as transcendent, devout, patriotic, and brave—plays a central role. The intentions of the sculptor and committee for the London memorial are made manifest by the fact that the viewer is given a great deal of textual guidance. The inscription refers to the manner of her death by recording the time, "Dawn," as well as the date and place of execution. In addition, "For King and Country" is engraved above the statue and the words "Humanity, Devotion, Fortitude, and Sacrifice" are found on each of the four sides in large letters. These textual clues guide the viewer to prioritize Cavell's martyrdom, her embodiment of humanity and civilization in the face of barbarism.

A comparable French vision of nursing as an idealized, feminized version of male military sacrifice, this time understood in terms of a Catholic conception of martyrdom, is found in the stained-glass windows of the memorial chapel at the national ossuary in Douaumont, painted and designed by Georges Desvallières in 1927. All of the windows in the chapel revolve around the theme of sacrifice and redemption, with two of them devoted to a nurse and a soldier who are presented as sainted martyrs, ascending to heaven in the arms of angels. Having converted to Catholicism in 1904, Desvallières vowed to produce only religious art after his son Daniel was killed in action at age nineteen in 1915. In 1919, he set up the Atelier d'art sacré, with painter Maurice Denis, with the aim of revitalizing religious art.[13] Male and female sacrifice embodied in the figures of soldier and nurse is also present in the frieze Desvallières painted for the private chapel of Jacques Rouché at Saint-Privat, which he completed in 1925. In *Dieu le père* (God the Father) (1920), Jesus holds a protecting cloak over a French soldier (modeled on Desvallières's dead son, Daniel) and nurse (modeled on Sabine, Desvallières's daughter) who kneel side by side, while the Virgin Mary welcomes them into heaven.[14] As Jean-Philippe Rey notes, in Desvallières's redemptive vision the idealized nurse–soldier couple becomes the joint representative of humanity: "The sacrifice of the soldiers becomes the remedy for sin. The communion of saints is restored, the chosen couple (*poilu* and nurse) intercedes on behalf of the inhabitants of the earth."[15]

Thus, while the nurses who appear on Roslyn's Darwen memorial and in Desvallières's religious art are placed within different conceptions of sacrifice—civic and religious—in both cases, the sexes are not placed in a hierarchical relationship, but side by side. Men and women, home and front, are understood as having been united by their suffering and by a collective spirit of sacrifice. The nurse's and the soldier's contributions are therefore presented as having some degree of equivalence and as metonymically standing in for the sacrifices made in wartime by a whole community.

NURSES REMEMBERING NURSES

The memorials that construct a vision of a community united in its collective sacrifice still distinguish, though, between the kinds of service carried out and sacrifices offered by men and by women. Nurses are praised for the way in which they extended their "devotion" and "humanity" beyond the home front to the front itself. They are presented as having acted out to the full a specifically female brand of service to their nation, supporting, nurturing, and healing the servicemen who are often designated symbolically as their sons or brothers. Other First World War memorials, however, and particularly those that commemorate nurses who were killed during the war, present women as female veterans, as more direct equivalents of dead servicemen.

While to some extent, like all commemorations, interwar memorials and ceremonies for nurses who had died in the war functioned as a focus for private grief, they were also vehicles for public messages about the nursing profession, and in particular about the value of nurses' contribution to the war. The commemorative discourse in these memorials combines private mourning with the public affirmation of the women's deaths as honorable war deaths, underlining the nursing organizations' sacrifices and devotion to the nation and thereby implicitly demanding public recognition and gratitude. An interesting French example of this kind of memorial to nurses was unveiled in 1923 after having been commissioned by one of the three organizations that made up the French Red Cross, the Union des Femmes de France (UFF). The sculptor was Berthe Girardet, who had volunteered for the UFF during the war and who produced several commemorative pieces in the interwar years.[16] It was unveiled in the headquarters of the UFF in Paris, and comprised a bas-relief featuring a group of nurses, with two plaques listing forty-eight members who had died. The bas-relief was described in the following terms during the commemoration ceremony by UFF President Mme Henri Galli, widow of the leader of the right-wing Ligue des Patriotes (League of Patriots): "With profound artistry fed by superior intelligence, and with religious sensibility, [Mme Girardet] has been able to reproduce the solemn dignity and the intense interior life exuded by these faces . . . which, as if they had haloes, have the character of religious icons."[17] These Red Cross nurses thus embraced, at least to some extent, dominant conceptions of nurses as transhistorical incarnations of saintly womanhood. The 1923 ceremony, however, equally functioned to shore up the identity of the Red Cross nurses as war veterans. Mme Galli's speech directly aligned the nurses' deaths with the "supreme sacrifice" made by soldiers:

> The emotions that bring us together today are sorrow and grief, but also pride, and we reverently pay homage to the memory of these valiant women who paid with their life for the fervent sense of altruism, heroic devotion and superior and patriotic virtues that they possessed. . . . Let the memory of the generosity of the nurses' lives that you grieve for . . . of the good that they did . . . and finally the memory that they too served France as her heroic defenders, that they carried out the noblest of missions, let these poignant memories relieve your suffering.[18]

The discourse here is familiar from unveiling ceremonies for soldiers that took place in every town and village in France and Britain in the years following the Armistice, in which the grieving audience was "urged to convert its grief to pride," except that the subjects of grief, gratitude, and glorification were women rather than male combatants.[19]

It is a discourse that was repeated in other commemorative activities for First World War nurses that took place in the interwar period. The newspaper article recounting the unveiling ceremony of the Irish Military Nurses' Memorial in Arbour Hill Garrison Chapel, Dublin, in 1921, was entitled "What Sacrifice May Teach," and the Reverend C. A. Peacocke's sermon, while praising the Irish nurses for "showing the highest qualities of womanhood," equally asked the congregation to "go away strengthened, helped and lifted up" after seeing in the memorial "a wonderful record of service, of character, of fortitude, of the highest and best gifts that God gave to man and woman."[20] The 1919 report by board member Colonel de Witt-Guizot on the activities of the Société de Secours aux Blessés militaires (SSBM) used more overtly military language and imagery when evoking the wartime deaths of the society's volunteer nurses:

> If I could I would invite you to stand, shout "Attention" and call for the playing of the Last Post. . . . To honor their memory I want the General Secretary to establish a "Roll of Honor" which, when read in schools and in family homes, will remind our children that French women spilled blood for them on the sacred ground of their homeland . . . and future generations will pass on their names, wreathed in glory.[21]

Many commemorations of female nurses who died on war service contained in this way a blend of traditional images of nurses as icons of womanhood with a discourse that set up their deaths as quasi-military sacrifices for the defense of the nation. During the 1921 service held for the unveiling of the Scottish Military Nurses War Memorial at St Giles' Cathedral, Edinburgh, Lieutenant-General Sir Francis Davis simultaneously praised the "sympathy and magic touch" of the nurses as "ministering angels," while stating that the memorial should serve as an example to future generations: "These ladies did not earn their crown in the day of battle. They earned it in the patient discharge of their duty, some killed by enemy action, victims of the malice of our foes."[22] Similarly, in France the local newspaper report of the unveiling of the Monument à la memoire des infirmières (Monument to the Memory of Nurses) in Berck-sur-Mer (Pas de Calais), instigated by local veterans and unveiled in 1924, recognized the "sublime role" and "unceasing devotion" of the nurses while emphasizing that they had "fallen on the field of honor" and noting that the ceremony ended with "the tricolor, the flag of glory and gratitude, that covered the monument being slowly raised."[23] The equation of nurses killed in the war with the male war dead is equally discernible in a statue designed by French sculptor Maxime

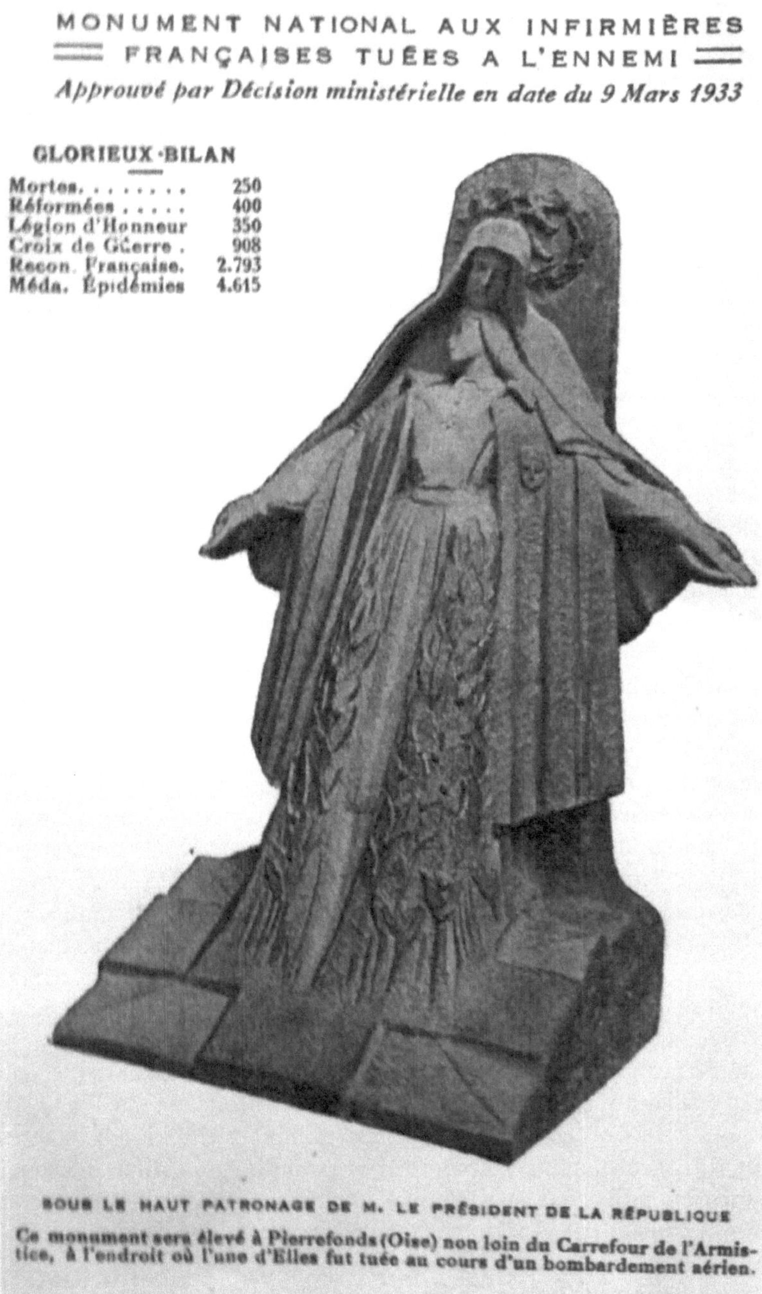

Figure A.3 Statue on the Monument national aux infirmières françaises tuées à l'ennemi, 1933, Pierrefonds (Oise). Fundraising pamphlet, Bibliothèque Marguerite Durand, Paris.

Réal del Sarte, a prolific nationalist sculptor of war memorials and Joan of Arc devotee, for the Monument national aux infirmières françaises tuées à l'ennemi (National Monument to French Nurses Killed in Action) in Pierrefonds (Oise), the committee for which had both veteran and nurse representation.[24] This 1933 statue featured an androgynous Pietà/Christ figure with outstretched arms supporting the body of a dead nurse, also with arms outstretched and who is dressed in medieval clothing reminiscent of Joan of Arc (Figure A.3). Its design reverses, in gender terms, many Pietàs that feature on French war memorials, including some examples by Réal del Sarte himself, in which the body of a French infantryman is presented, Christ-like, with outstretched arms, and is supported in the protective embrace of a Mary or Joan of Arc figure.[25]

While military authorities and veterans tended to prioritize transcendent feminine virtues in memorials to nurses killed in the war, nursing organizations themselves tended to place the emphasis more on the challenging conditions and risks to life and health of wartime nursing in a bid to underscore the value of their service to the state. This is particularly true of British trained nurses. In 1922, the British Military Nurses Memorial Committee, chaired by Matron-in-Chief Sarah Oram, commissioned a statue for St Paul's Cathedral by sculptor Benjamin Clemens entitled "Bombed" (that was ultimately not accepted by the cathedral authorities due to lack of space), a commission that suggests a desire for a representation of nursing work that emphasized frontline risk.[26] The sculpted figures on the military nurses' memorial in St Giles' Cathedral, Edinburgh, are also interesting in terms of the meanings with which they are charged. The classical female figure on the left is kneeling, her head bowed, carrying a wreath, while on the right another holds her head upright and, warrior-like, carries a flag in one hand and a dagger in the other (Figure A.4). Above the statues are a list of the Scottish members of the QAIMNS and QAIMNSR who died in the war. The figures are described as representing "Grief and Sacrifice" and "Courage and Patriotism," and thus the iconography of this memorial points to the dual role of the nurses, as both mourners paying tribute to their lost colleagues and the soldiers they nursed and as active participants who risked death.[27]

The French Monument à la gloire des infirmières françaises et alliées victimes de leur dévouement (Monument to the Glory of French and Allied Nurses, Victims of Their Devotion) also combines traditional imagery of nurses with elements underlining their quasi-military sacrifice. This memorial, unveiled in Rheims in 1924, had a committee presided over by eighty-eight-year-old Juliette Adam, well-known feminist and *femme du monde* who had converted to Catholicism in the early 1900s.[28] The committee also included both doctors and professional nurses. The iconography of Denys Puech's sculpture reinvokes the Catholic-inspired French vision of nurses as grieving Pietàs over the dead Christ/poilu. If the figures place the nurse in a familiar position of idealized maternal devotion, however, the

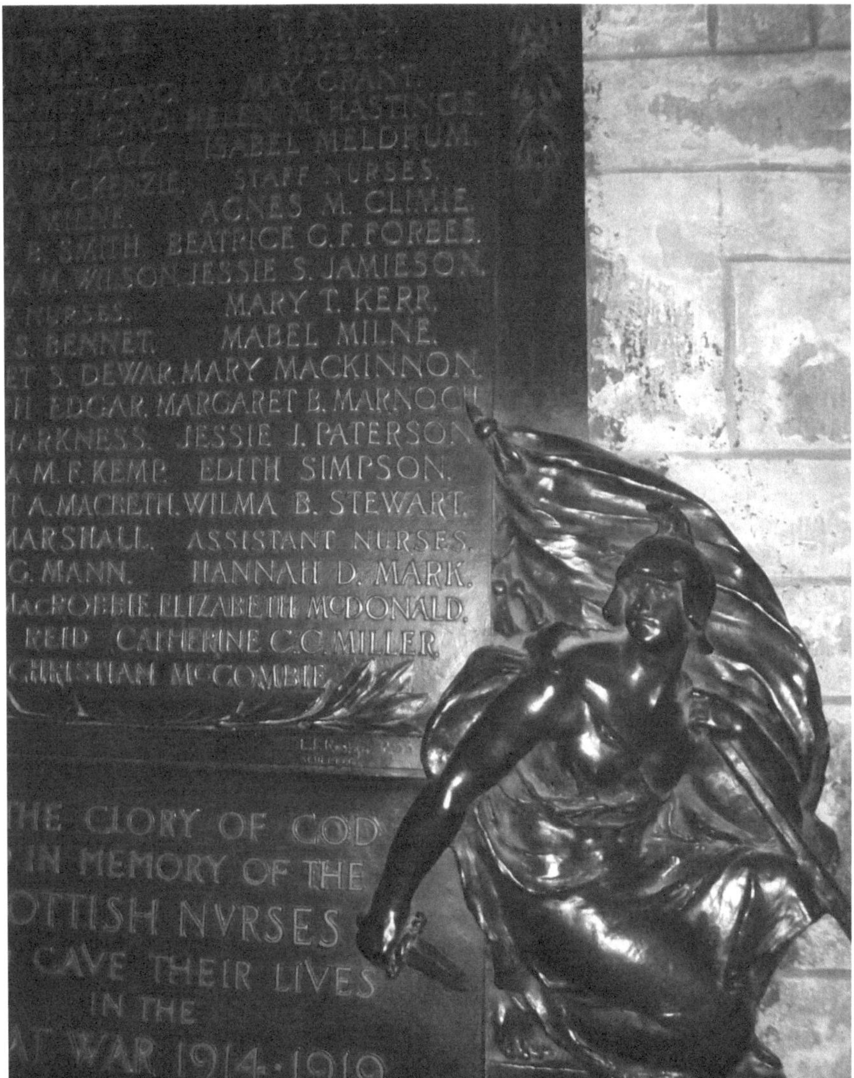

Figure A.4 Detail of memorial plaque, 1921, sculpted by Louis Roslyn, St Giles' Cathedral, Edinburgh. Photograph by author.

memorial's inscription comes closer to aligning the work of nurses with that of the soldiers: "On land and sea, they shared the soldier's dangers. They braved, in shelled and torpedoed hospitals, enemy fire, contagion and exhaustion. In relieving suffering, they aided victory. Let us honor them.

They will forever live in the memory of their proud and grateful nations." The design and inscription were undoubtedly influenced by the sentiments of the committee's chair, Juliette Adam, reflecting her religious faith and her fervent patriotism as well as her continued support for women's rights. The genesis of the Rheims nurses' memorial was not only sparked by grief, but by the committee's desire to express publicly a combination of religious, nationalist, and feminist beliefs.

Thus, while Adam's speech drew on traditional understandings of nurses' "feminine" virtues, describing the "courageous devotion" of the "heroic victims," she was equally keen to underscore the value of women's contribution and sacrifice to the Allied nations.[29] One way in which the latter was done was through the compilation of a "Livre d'or" (Roll of Honor) listing 979 names of Allied nurses who died in France, with an accompanying inscription on the monument stating that "the town of Rheims will faithfully keep in its archives the Roll of Honor of these noble women who fell on the field of honor."[30] Thomas Laqueur has argued that the extensive naming of the dead of the First World War, particularly significant for the hundreds of thousands of cases of missing soldiers' bodies, was "an enormous and unprecedented part of . . . the memorials of the war." Naming a soldier (and especially a private who might normally have expected to be buried anonymously in a common grave) was to individualize, to commemorate, and to dignify him without necessarily limiting the meaning of his death to a specific "cause"; to resort, in Laqueur's words, "to a sort of commemorative hyper-nominalism."[31] Recording, inscribing, and sacralizing the names of nurses who had died as a result of war service was thus a way of integrating their deaths into the mainstream of First World War commemoration. In the case of the Rheims monument, other officials followed Adam's lead and embraced her categorization of the nurses as "mort[es] pour la France." M. Mennecier, Sub Prefect of Rheims, for example, declared "on behalf of the government" in his speech that:

> Today, perhaps for the first time, but forever more, we will proclaim together in front of this monument, illuminated like other monuments by the glory of sacrifice, that it is right and necessary to unite in our gratitude, as they have already been united in immortality, the names of soldiers killed in action with the names of these admirable nurses who also, and in their thousands, responded to the call to arms, risked life and limb in order to carry out their duties.[32]

Thus, while the iconography of the Rheims memorial to Allied nurses positioned them as "ministering angels," the Roll of Honor and other inscriptions placed their deaths overtly within the framework of military commemoration.

In giving the nurses who were killed in the conflict the status of fallen combatants, the nursing organizations were, on the one hand, attempting to comfort bereaved families, and, on the other, making public, political gestures. Judith Butler has argued in relation to the commemoration of the 9/11 terrorist attacks in New York that "the obituary functions as the instrument by which grievability is publicly distributed. It is the means by which a life becomes, or fails to become, a publicly grievable life, an icon for national self-recognition, the means by which a life becomes noteworthy."[33] This insight is relevant to the interwar context in which certain individuals and organizations were claiming lost female lives as publicly grievable sacrifices for the nation. Although nurses' memorials were in part motivated by private grief for lost members, nurses' organizations also used the opportunity offered by the prestige of nursing in the discourse of commemoration for political ends, for example, to add weight to their struggle for professionalization. In commemorating nurses who had died, they were also, implicitly, demanding gratitude and greater recognition of the value of all nurses' wartime service to the state.

REMEMBERING THE FIRST WORLD WAR NURSE IN POPULAR CULTURE

Whereas in the 1920s nurses were often portrayed as having some degree of equivalence to mobilized men, especially those nurses who had died on active service, attitudes evolved in the 1930s, mapping the evolution of attitudes toward the war more generally. Janet Watson notes in relation to Britain that from the late 1920s onward, as the "disillusionment" narratives of pacifist veteran-writers and poets took hold of the public imagination, "women war workers . . . shifted from the separate-but-parallel peers of their brothers-in-arms to something so different that comparison between the two groups was no longer conceivable."[34] Women's war stories that did not focus on the horrors and suffering of the trenches were effectively sidelined, and antiwar narratives penned by male veterans tended to dominate public memory of the war on both sides of the Channel. From the 1930s onward, in other words, a national "War Story" took root in both nations in which young soldiers "were led to early and ghastly deaths in muddy wastes by incompetent generals for reasons that were seemingly futile."[35] It was a story in which nurses had only a minor bit-part.

However, this changed in the context of second-wave feminist rediscovery of women's voices from the Great War that took place from the late 1970s onward. In Britain, this was particularly evident in two landmark cultural events: the Imperial War Museum's *Women at War* exhibition that ran from November 1977 to January 1978, and the republication and television dramatization of former VAD Vera Brittain's 1933 memoir *Testament of Youth*. The Imperial War Museum's exhibition was accompanied by the publication of Arthur Marwick's lavishly illustrated book *Women at War 1914–1918*.[36] Both were influential in educating the public about women's diverse roles during the conflict, and they highlighted nursing as one of women's most important wartime activities. Marwick's chronicle attempted to include the experience of ordinary women as well as that of exceptional "heroines," which had been the focus of David Mitchell's more celebratory 1966 study, *Women on the War Path*.[37] Focusing on the variety of women's wartime activities, *Women at War* argued that the war had opened doors for women, effectively improving their social status. The conclusions of Marwick's book were subsequently challenged by several historians, who argued that women's progress in terms, for example, of employment rights was both limited and temporary.[38] Both the book and the exhibition reproduced the photographs compiled for the Imperial War Museum's *Women at Work* collection in 1917–1918 somewhat uncritically, not analyzing the extent to which the photographs had been used for the government promotion of female wartime employment.[39] Moreover, Marwick helped to cement two popular conceptions of First World War nursing that have persisted: first, he focused more on the complaints and experiences of VADs than on those of trained nurses and, second, he presented nursing as a means of escaping the limitations of prewar domesticity, underplaying the extent to which many professional nurses, and some volunteers, had been active in the public sphere long before 1914.[40]

This vision of war nursing as both liberating and empowering also influenced the writings of some feminist literary critics in the 1980s and 1990s. A common argument, drawing on interwar literary sources, suggested that while the war left men emasculated, it gave women, including nurses, a degree of matriarchal power over men. The most commonly cited critic who expounded this argument is Sandra Gilbert. Her discussion of the representation of nurses in certain wartime novels, for example, presents their hospital work as a kind of weapon in the "battle of the sexes." "The figure of the nurse ultimately takes on a majesty which hints that she is mistress rather than slave, goddess rather than supplicant. After all, when men are immobilized and dehumanized, it is only these women who possess the (matriarchal) formulas for survival."[41] It was not only in literary, cultural, or historical studies, however, that the understanding of nursing work in these terms had currency. In Britain, the notion of wartime nursing as "empowering" for women was further embedded in popular consciousness by the renewed success and wide dissemination of Vera Brittain's war story in the 1970s and 1980s. Although to some extent she had an atypical experience, Brittain has become shorthand not only for First World War nursing, but for women's experiences of the war more generally. Her first volume of autobiography, *Testament of Youth*, was republished in paperback by Virago in 1978 and swiftly became a best seller, assisted by its adaptation into a BBC drama series in 1979.[42] Indeed, her story continues to attract attention, having been the subject of a recent BBC docudrama narrated by the comedian Jo Brand.[43] Its ongoing influence can also be seen in the fact that, as Dan Todman notes, "In two thirds of the novels [about the war] produced in the period from 1978 to 1998, the principal activity for the main female characters was nursing, usually in France as a VAD."[44] A comparison of Brittain's wartime diaries with her published memoirs reveal the extent to which she rewrote her war story in the early 1930s in order to conform to the generic expectations of contemporary male antiwar tales of loss, horror, and disillusionment.[45] Yet what was often retained and reproduced in the popular fiction that followed in its wake was an exciting tale of female empowerment in which the war brought about a watershed for women. Somewhat paradoxically, then, Brittain's pacifist narrative, in which her narrator functions as a grief-stricken harbinger of doom, as a spokesperson for a generation who had lived through a war that should never be repeated, was often reread in the 1970s and 1980s as a feminist chronicle of war as an escape route from a cloistered and patriarchal bourgeois lifestyle.

France has also seen a renewal of interest in women's war experiences, although not to the same extent as in Britain. Women's roles in 1914–1918 have been somewhat overshadowed by the concentration by historians, writers, and filmmakers on women's roles under German occupation in the Second World War, in which the figure of the female resistance heroine dominates. However, in the literary and cinematic representations of the First World War that have proliferated since the 1990s, the nurse has remained an essential ingredient. A key French example is that of the 2001 film *La Chambre des officiers* (The Officer's Ward), directed by François Dupeyron, which achieved international box-office and critical success. In Dupeyron's film, both central female characters are nurses, and they embody the two versions of the wartime nurse that have persisted in the popular imagination. The middle-aged Anaïs is a selfless, maternal "white angel" (the nickname given to nurses in France) who helps to heal officer Adrien's physical and psychological scars. Her character is close, in effect, to the idealized images to be found in wartime propaganda, as well as to the nurse-as-sanctuary figure that features in many male-authored interwar combat novels.[46] In contrast, Marguerite, a young former nurse who is a fellow *gueule cassée* (facially injured patient) for hero Adrien, is condemned by the patriarchal double standards of her bourgeois family, who see her as unmarriageable as a result of her facial injuries and therefore as worthless. She is thus representative of recent feminist revisionist interpretations of women's wartime roles, in that her character both blurs the line between combatant and noncombatant and implies that the war led middle-class women to reject the limitations of prewar gender norms.

Two examples from books published in Britain and France to accompany more recent museum exhibitions focusing on women and the First World War illustrate the persistence of a focus on war nursing as a liberating activity for middle- or upper-class women. The chapter on First World War nursing in Kate Adie's 2003 book *Corsets to Camouflage*, which was published to coincide with a 2003–2004 Imperial War Museum exhibition entitled *Women and War*, mentions both trained and untrained nurses, but her case studies are mostly well-known British middle- or upper-class volunteers, reproducing photographs of Elsie Knocker and Mairi Chisholm, the Duchesses of Westminster and Sutherland, and Mabel St Clair Stobart. She is also clearly influenced by interpretations of women's war service as liberating from dominant gender imperatives, arguing that "from a world of tennis parties and tedious small-talk, respectability and the pursuit of a suitable marriage, thousands of women proved quietly and doggedly that they could see the worst of war and deal with it."[47] In France, a 2010–2011 exhibition in the newly opened Musée de la Grande Guerre (Museum of the Great War) in Meaux, near Paris, also played on the popular notion of sheltered young ladies looking for escape and adventure: "This desire to be useful attracted idle young women from wealthy families who all rushed to undertake nursing training courses from mid-August 1913."[48]

Of course, there were some middle- and upper-class French and British women for whom wartime nursing constituted a transformative first venture out of the domestic sphere. But an undue emphasis on the "adventures" of wealthy volunteer nurses has distorted the overall picture of First World War nursing. As in the interwar period, museums, Internet sites, and television programs rarely focus on trained nurses, military nurses, female doctors, male nurses and orderlies, or women who worked in theaters other than the western front. The emphasis tends still to be on young volunteers rather than on the thousands of older women who were already active in the public sphere, whether in paid or voluntary work, and who simply transferred their skills into a wartime context. As Gail Braybon reminds us, "women's wartime history was, and often still is, overlaid with myth," and this is especially true in the case of First World War nursing.[49] As the centenary of the First World War approaches, these myths continue to be recycled in popular representations of the conflict. Yet, as the contributions to this volume have shown, the analysis of a wider range of sources, such as the letters and memoirs of trained professionals, offers us a broader perspective. Equally, the revisiting of better-known nursing memoirs, such as those produced by Americans Mary Borden and Ellen La Motte, reveals that the common trope of a wealthy young volunteer nurse whose story can be easily mapped onto the "disillusionment" narrative dominant in the 1930s, or read as a liberating release from stifling domesticity, also demands reevaluation. Rather, the memoirs, letters, and diaries that have been analyzed here show that witnessing the war as a nurse was a complex and sometimes conflictual role for women. It required the simultaneous adoption of different, sometimes clashing, perspectives: nurses were observers of suffering, active participants in the war effort, professional carers, and stand-ins for a male patient's mother, sister, or lover. The nurses whose voices are quoted in this volume often express both a sense of pride in their ability to carry out these roles well and a sense of unease about the ways in which these multiple roles were not always compatible. Yet it is precisely the extent to which nurses often functioned as a kind of bridge or conduit between front and home front, between combatant and noncombatant, that makes their shifting perspectives so important an addition to the study of the First World War.

NOTES

1. J. Watson, "Khaki Girls, VADs, and Tommy's Sisters: Gender and Class in First World War Britain," *International History Review* 13, no. 1 (1997): 33–35.
2. Letter from an anonymous military nurse using the pseudonym "Après la guerre," *Times* (18 August 1919).
3. On women as mourners in First World War memorials and ceremonies, see A. Becker, *Les Monuments aux morts: Mémoire de la Grande Guerre* (Paris: Errance, 1989); Grayzel, *Women's Identities at War*; A. King, *Memorials of the Great War in Britain: The Symbolism and Politics of Remembrance* (Oxford: Berg, 1998); C. Moriarty, "Private Grief and Public Remembrance: British First World War Memorials," in *War and Memory in the Twentieth Century*, ed. M. Evans and K. Lunn (Oxford, Berg: 1997), 125–42; D. Sherman, *The Construction of Memory in Interwar France* (Chicago: University of Chicago Press, 1999).
4. Kathryn McPherson notes in this context that "[Nurses'] presence in the public space, whether in their daily work or in memorials, did not fundamentally challenge prevailing perceptions of appropriate femininity"; see K. McPherson, "Carving Out a Past: The Canadian Nurses' Association War Memorial," *Histoire sociale/Social History* 29 (1996): 419.
5. A. Becker, "From Death to Memory: The National Ossuaries in France after the Great War," *History and Memory* 5 (1993): 32. See also A. Becker, *La Guerre et la foi: De la mort à la mémoire* (Paris: Armand Colin, 1994), 122.
6. Archives départementales de la Loire, article accompanying the 2008 exhibition *La Loire au service des blessés.*
7. Roslyn sculpted a similar monument at Blackley, Greater Manchester, with four figures holding emblems representing the army, navy, air force, and nursing services (since removed) that was unveiled in 1921. There was also a proposal by the mayor of Oxford for a design including "four figures in bronze [. . .] an infantry soldier, a gunner, a yeoman, and a nurse" (*Observer*, 2 May 1920). The Oxford War Memorial Committee, however, eventually chose the design by John Thorpe, Gilbert Gardner, and Thomas Rayson.
8. For details of Cavell's role in organizing an escape network for Allied soldiers, see K. Pickles, *Transnational Outrage: The Death and Commemoration of Edith Cavell* (Basingstoke: Palgrave, 2005).
9. 1 February 1916, quoted in G. Bresc-Bautier and A. Pingeot, *Sculptures des jardins du Louvre, du Carrousel et des Tuileries* (Paris: Editions de la Réunion des musées nationaux, 1986), 2,360. The committee was presided over by Paul Painlevé, Minister of Education, who had written a panegyric to Cavell in 1915. See P. Painlevé, "Introduction," in *La Vie et la mort de Miss Edith Cavell*, by Anonymous (Paris: Fontemoing et cie., 1915), x–xi. The models of other entries show similar interpretations, although interestingly the design placed second, sculpted by André Vermare, has a classically draped Cavell standing defiantly, gazing toward the horizon with a much smaller French soldier and nurse seated on either side of her, a version

of Cavell that resembles the London memorial. See *Le Pays de France* (9 November 1916).

10. *Le Figaro* (13 June 1920).
11. C. Sniter, "La gloire des femmes célèbres: Métamorphoses et disparité de la statuaire publique parisienne de 1870 à nos jours," *Sociétés et Représentations* 26 (2008): 153–70.
12. S. Malvern, "'For King and Country': Frampton's Edith Cavell (1915–1920) and the Writing of Gender in Memorials to the Great War,' in *Sculpture and the Pursuit of a Modern Ideal in Britain, 1880–1930*, ed. D. Getsy (Aldershot: Ashgate, 2004), 221; Pickles, *Transnational Outrage*, 120.
13. Desvallières also frequently painted the *poilu* as Christ in reimaginings of the Way of the Cross, such as the murals depicting the soldier's "way of the Cross" at the Catholic housing project in the fourteenth arrondissement of Paris. Becker, *La Guerre*, 130–31; Winter, *Sites of Memory*, 53.
14. C. Racine, "Le mot à l'œuvre dans le décor peint de la chapelle de Jacques Rouché à Saint-Privat par Georges Desvallières (1919–1924)," unpublished conference presentation at "Le Mot à l'oeuvre" conference, 16 June 2009, Institut National de l'Histoire de l'Art, Paris; C. Ambroselli, "Georges Desvallières. Les grands élans de l'âme, de l'esprit et du cœur," in *Georges Desvallières et le Salon d'Automne*, ed. C. Ambroselli (Paris: Somogy, 2003), 36. Sabine Desvallières became a nun in 1926, taking the name Marie de la Grâce, and died in 1935.
15. J. P. Rey, "Desvallières et la guerre de 1914–1918," *Société de l'histoire de l'art français* (1988): 197–211, quoted in Becker, *La Guerre*, 131.
16. Berthe Girardet was a Swiss-born sculptor and wife of the engraver Paul Girardet, whose son, Jean-Paul Girardet, an architect turned pilot, was killed in a flying accident in 1917. Like Desvallières, Girardet produced sculpture that interpreted the losses of the war within a Catholic framework of suffering, sacrifice, and redemption. Her works included *A l'hôpital pendant la Grande Guerre* (1919) and *Aux héros inconnus*, featuring a mourning female figure, that was exhibited in the Ossuaire at Douaumont in 1923. Placed on a classical pedestal and wreathed in victory laurels, a veiled Virgin holds her fingers to her lips, suggesting the need for respect, silence, and resignation.
17. *Bulletin mensuel de l'Union des Femmes de France* (1 January 1923): 9.
18. Ibid., 7.
19. Moriarty, "Private Grief and Public Remembrance," 135.
20. *Irish Times* (7 November 1921). Cutting in TNA, WO 222/2135.
21. Croix Rouge Française, *Assemblée générale du 23 novembre 1919 de la Société de Secours aux Blessés Militaires: Rapport du Colonel de Witt-Guizot.*
22. *Glasgow Herald* (4 November 1921). Cutting in TNA, WO222/2135.
23. *L'Echo de Paris* (24 November 1924).
24. The text on the 1933 fundraising leaflet for this memorial also combined traditional images of nurses as "animated by altruism and reminding poilus, by their gentleness and their self-abnegation, of a mother, wife or sister," with a direct alignment to dead soldiers. "In this vast, pious homage to combatants killed in action no memorials remember the heroic sacrifice of our nurses" (Bibliothèque Marguerite Durand, DOS Infirmière militaire).
25. See, for example, Réal del Sarte's Pietà on the Monument du 106e régiment, Les Eparges. Reproduced in M. Hurcombe, "Raising the Dead: Visual Representations of the Combatant's Body in Interwar France," *Journal of War and Culture Studies* 1, no. 2 (2008): 169.
26. Minutes of the Military Nurses Memorial Committee, 23 June 1922, TNA, WO 222/2135. Benjamin Clemens sculpted the realist bronze pieces *St.*

John's Ambulance Bearers in 1919 and *VAD Worker* in 1920, which no doubt had been seen by the committee.

27. *Nursing Mirror and Midwives Journal* (12 November 1921): 121.
28. Juliette Adam published an early feminist text, *Les Idées antiproudhoniennes*, in 1858 and remained an active suffragist all her life. She published *Chrétienne* in 1913 (after having published *Païenne* in 1883), publicly announcing her conversion to Catholicism. Throughout the war she devoted herself to the war effort, helping to fundraise for charities aimed at helping soldiers and founding *Le Journal des Poilus*. She continued to write articles attacking Germany as she had done since the Franco-Prussian war, but also published in 1919 *La Vie des âmes*, expressing her horror at the loss of life. See A. Hogenhuis-Seliverstoff, *Juliette Adam* (Paris: L'Harmattan, 2001).
29. *Bulletin mensuel de l'Union des Femmes de France* (1 February 1925): 29.
30. These were originally deposited in the Red Cross archives in Rheims but were transferred to Rheims municipal archives in 2005.
31. T. W. Laqueur, "Memory and Naming in the Great War," in *Commemorations: The Politics of National Identity*, ed. J. R. Gillis (Princeton, NJ: Princeton University Press, 1994), 164, 160.
32. *Bulletin mensuel de l'Union des Femmes de France* (1 February 1925): 30.
33. J. Butler, *Precarious Life: The Power of Mourning and Violence* (London: Verso, 2004), 34.
34. Watson, *Fighting Different Wars*, 264.
35. H. Strachan, *The First World War* (London: Simon and Schuster, 2003), inside flap.
36. Marwick, *Women at War.*
37. D. Mitchell, *Women on the War Path: The Story of the Women of the First World War* (London: Cape, 1966).
38. See in particular D. Thom, *Nice Girls and Rude Girls: Women Workers in World War I* (London: I. B. Tauris, 1998); and G. Braybon, *Women Workers in the First World War* (London: Croom Helm, 1981).
39. See G. Braybon, "Winners or Losers: Women's Role in the War Story," in *Evidence, History and the Great War: Historians and the Impact of 1914–1918*, ed. G. Braybon (Oxford: Berghahn, 2003), 86–112.
40. Watson, *Fighting Different Wars*, 284.
41. S. M. Gilbert, "Literary Men, Literary Women and the Great War," in *Behind the Lines: Gender and the Two World Wars*, ed. M. R. Higonnet, J. Jenson, S. Michel, and M. Collins Weitz (New Haven and London: Yale University Press, 1987), 211.
42. Paul Berry and Mark Bostridge remark in their 1995 biography of Brittain that sales in Britain alone of *Testament of Youth* amounted to "close to three-quarters of a million." P. Berry and M. Bostridge, *Vera Brittain: A Life* (London: Chatto, 1995), 2.
43. *A Woman in Love and War: Vera Brittain*, first broadcast on BBC 2, 9 November 2008.
44. D. Todman, *The Great War: Myth and Memory* (London: Hambledon Continuum, 2005), 183.
45. Watson, *Fighting Different Wars*, 248–55.
46. Françoise Thébaud notes, for example, the interwar reoccurrence of the "myth of woman as salvation and consolation." F. Thébaud, "La Grande Guerre," in *Histoire des femmes en occident 5: Le XXe siècle*, ed. G. Duby (Paris: Plon, 1992), 43.
47. K. Adie, *Corsets to Camouflage: Women and War* (London: Hodder and Stoughton, 2003), 76, 80.

48. Catalogue for the exhibition entitled *1914–1918: Les femmes dans la Grande Guerre*, Musée de la Grande Guerre, 11 November 2010–31 March 2011.
49. G. Braybon, ed., *Evidence, History and the Great War,* 88.

Bibliography

ARCHIVES CONSULTED

Australian War Memorial, Canberra, Australia
Brittain Archives, William Ready Collection, McMaster University, US
Churchill College Archive, Cambridge, UK
Imperial War Museum, London, UK
J. S. Battye Library of West Australian History, Australia
Library and Archives Canada, Ottawa, Ontario, Canada
Liddle Collection, Brotherton Library, University of Leeds, UK
Mitchell Library, Australia
The National Archives, Kew, UK
Red Cross Archives, London, UK
Rheims Municipal Archives, France
Royal College of Nursing Archives, Edinburgh, UK
State Library of Victoria, Australia
Wellcome Trust Library and Archives, UK

PUBLISHED SOURCES

Abel-Smith, B. *A History of the Nursing Profession*. London: William Heinemann, 1960.

Abrams, S. "Go Down to Suffering and Raise It Up." *Public Health Nursing* 28, no. 1 (2010): 103–4.

Acton, C. "Diverting the Gaze: The Unseen Text in Women's War Writing." *College Literature* 31, no. 2 (2004): 53–79.

Acton, C. *Grief in Wartime: Private Pain, Public Discourse*. Basingstoke: Palgrave MacMillan, 2007.

Adam-Smith, P. *The Anzacs*. Melbourne: Thomas Nelson Australia Pty, 1978.

Adam-Smith, P. *Australian Women at War*. Melbourne: Thomas Nelson Australia, 1984.

Adie, K. *Corsets to Camouflage: Women and War*. London: Hodder and Stoughton, 2003.

Alesson, J. *Les Femmes décorées de la légion d'honneur et les femmes militaires*. Paris: G. Melet libraire-éditeur, 1886.

Ambert, Général J. *Gaulois et Germains: Récits militaires*, 4 vols. Paris: Bloud et Barral, 1883–1885.

Ambroselli, C. "Georges Desvallières. Les grands élans de l'âme, de l'esprit et du cœur," in *Georges Desvallières et le Salon d'Automne*, ed. C. Ambroselli. Paris: Somogy, 2003.

Ambrosius, L. E. "Woodrow Wilson and George W. Bush: Historical Comparisons of Ends and Means in Their Foreign Policies." *Diplomatic History* 30, no. 3 (2006): 509–43.

Anonymous. *An American VAD, Letters from Two Hospitals*. Boston: Atlantic Monthly Press, 1919.

Anonymous. "The Australian War-Nurse." *Sydney Morning Herald* (27 June 1917): 5.

Anonymous. "Cent neuf femmes légionnaires." *La Vie heureuse* (December 1905).

Anonymous. *Diary of a Nursing Sister on the Western Front 1914–1915*. Edinburgh: William Blackwood and Sons, 1915.

Anonymous. "Editorial: Emotional Nursing." *British Journal of Nursing* 53 (19 December 1914): 357.

Anonymous. "Editorial: Tinsel Glory." *British Journal of Nursing* 53 (14 November 1914): 377.

Anonymous. "Is It Just?" in "Letters to the Editor." *British Journal of Nursing* 53 (4 July 1914): 22.

Anonymous. "La Cornette protectrice des blessés: Sœur Julie de Gerbéviller." *Lectures pour tous* (15 January 1916).

Anonymous. "L'Ambulance du Théâtre-Française." *L'Illustration* (21 January 1871): 35.

Anonymous. "Letter from Sister Bisset." *Una* (29 January 1916): 346.

Anonymous. "Letters to the Editor." *British Journal of Nursing* 53 (19 December 1914): 497.

Anonymous. *"Mademoiselle Miss": Letters from an American Girl Serving with the Rank of Lieutenant in a French Army Hospital at the Front*. Boston: W. A. Butterfield, 1916.

Anonymous. "The Nursing Outlook: War Fever and the War Spirit." *Nursing Mirror and Midwives Journal* 19 (22 August 1914): 397.

Anonymous. "Our Sisters." *Una* (28 February 1919): 383.

Anonymous. "Pour soigner les blessés militaires: Appel aux femmes." *Le Petit Parisien* (6 August 1914).

Anonymous. *President Wilson's Great Speeches and Other History Making Documents*. Chicago: Stanton and Van Vliet Co., 1919.

Anonymous. "Quelques exploits." *Echo de Paris* (27 December 1914).

Anonymous. *Report of the Committee on Alleged German Outrages Appointed by His Britannic Majesty's Government and Presided over by the Right Hon. Viscount Bryce*. London: H .M. Stationery Office, 1915.

Anonymous. "Visite d'un journaliste parisien." *Le Petit Parisien* (29 September 1914).

Antliff, M., and P. Leighten. *Cubism and Culture*. New York: Thames and Hudson, 2001.

Arnaud, L., and P. Bonnette. *La Femme sur le champ de bataille*. Paris: Henri Charles-Lavauzelle, 1912.

Atherton, G. *Life in the War Zone*. New York: New York Times, 1916.

Austin, S., and R. Austin. *The Body Snatchers: The History of the 3rd Australian Field Ambulance 1914–1918*. Rosebud, Victoria: Slouch Hat Publications, 1995.

Bagnold, E. *Diary without Dates*. London: Virago, 1978 [1918].

Bagnold, E. *Enid Bagnold's Autobiography*, Introduction by B. Willard. London: Century Publishing, 1985 [1969].

Bakhtin, M. *The Dialogic Imagination. Four Essays.* Trans. C. Emerson and M. Holquist. Austin: University of Texas Press, 1981.
Barker, M. *Nightingales in the Mud: The Digger Sisters of the Great War 1914–1918.* Sydney: Allen and Unwin, 1989.
Barrès, M. "L'âme des ruines." *Echo de Paris* (4 November 1914).
Barrett, J. W., and P. E. Deane. *The Australian Army Medical Corps in Egypt.* London: H. K. Lewis and Co., 1918.
Barton, E. C. *Hints to VAD Members in Hospitals, Approved by the Joint War Committee of the British Red Cross Society and the St. John Ambulance Association.* London: Nursing Times, Macmillan and Co., 1915.
Bashford, A. *Purity and Pollution: Gender, Embodiment and Victorian Medicine.* Basingstoke: Macmillan, 1998.
Bassett, J. *Guns and Brooches: Australian Army Nursing from the Boer War to the Gulf War.* Melbourne: Oxford University Press Australia, 1992.
Bateson, G. *Steps to an Ecology of Mind: Collected Essays in Anthropology, Psychiatry, Evolution and Epistemology.* Northvale, NJ: Jason Aronson, 1987.
Bean, C. E. W. *The Official History of Australia in the War of 1914–1918.* Vol. 2. Sydney: Angus and Robertson, 1941.
Beck, J. M. *The War and Humanity: A Further Discussion of the Ethics of the World War and the Attitude and Duty of the United States.* New York: G. P. Putnam's Sons, 1917.
Becker, A. "The Avant-Garde, Madness and the Great War." *Journal of Contemporary History* 35, no. 1 (2000): 71–84.
Becker, A. "From Death to Memory: The National Ossuaries in France after the Great War." *History and Memory* 5 (1993): 32–49.
Becker, A. *La Guerre et la foi: De la mort à la mémoire.* Paris: Armand Colin, 1994.
Becker, A. *Les Monuments aux morts: Mémoire de la Grande Guerre.* Paris: Errance, 1989.
Begg, R. Campbell. *Surgery on Trestles.* Norwich: Jarrold and Sons, 1967.
Bendall, E., and E. Raybould. *A History of the General Nursing Council 1919–1969.* London: GNC, 1969.
Benson, K. "Archival Analysis of the Committee on Public Information: The Relationship between Propaganda, Journalism and Popular Culture." *International Journal of Technology, Knowledge and Society* 6, no. 4 (2010): 151–64.
Bentley, N. "Museum Realism," in *Cambridge History of American Literature,* vol. 3. Cambridge: Cambridge University Press, 2005.
Bernhardt, S. *Ma double vie: mémoires de Sarah Bernhardt.* Paris: Charpentier et Fasquelle, 1907.
Berry, P., and M. Bostridge. *Vera Brittain: A Life.* London: Pimlico, 1995.
Bhabha, H. K. *Nation and Narration.* London: Routledge, 1990.
Binot, J.-M. *Héroïnes de la Grande Guerre.* Paris: Fayard, 2008.
Bishop, A., and M. Bostridge, eds. *Letters from a Lost Generation.* London: Little, Brown and Company, 1998.
Black, E. Walker. *Hospital Heroes.* New York: Charles Scribner's Sons, 1919.
Blunden, E. *Undertones of War.* Chicago: University of Chicago Press, 2007 [1928].
Borden, M. *The Forbidden Zone.* London: Heinemann, 1929.
Borden, M. *The Forbidden Zone.* Ed. H. Hutchison. London: Hesperus Press, 2008.
Borden, M. *Journey down a Blind Alley.* London: Hutchinson, 1946.
Borden-Turner, M. "At the Somme." *English Review* (August 1917).
Bouloumié, Dr. P. *Union des Femmes de France, conférence à Lyon le 3 avril 1886.* Paris: Coopération typographique, 1886.

Bourdieu, P. *Distinction: A Social Critique of the Judgement of Taste.* London: Routledge, 1984.
Bourke, J. *Dismembering the Male: Men's Bodies, Britain and the Great War.* Chicago: University of Chicago Press, 1996.
Bowser, T. *The Story of British VAD Work in the Great War.* London: Imperial War Museum, 2003; facsimile of the 1917 edition.
Braga, S. *Anzac Doctor: The Life of Sir Neville Howse, Australia's First VC.* Alexandria, NSW: Hale and Iremonger, 2000.
Braybon, G. "Winners or Losers: Women's Role in the War Story," in *Evidence, History and the Great War: Historians and the Impact of 1914–1918*, ed. G. Braybon, 125–42. Oxford: Berghahn, 2003.
Braybon, G. *Women Workers in the First World War.* London: Croom Helm, 1981.
Bresc-Bautier, G., and A. Pingeot. *Sculptures des jardins du Louvre, du Carrousel et des Tuileries.* Vol. 2. Paris: Editions de la Réunion des musées nationaux, 1986.
Brittain, V. *Testament of Youth.* Glasgow: Collins and Sons, 1980 [1933].
Brittain, V. *Verses of a V.A.D.* Foreword by M. C. Leighton. London: E. Macdonald, 1918.
Brothers, C. *War and Photography: A Cultural History.* London: Routledge, 1997.
Bucur, M. "Women's Stories as Sites of Memory: Gender and Remembering Romania's World Wars," in *Gender and War in Twentieth-Century Eastern Europe*, ed. N. M. Wingfield and M. Bucur, 171–92. Bloomington: Indiana University Press, 2006.
Bush, J. *Edwardian Ladies and Imperial Power.* London: University of Leicester Press, 2000.
Butler, A. G. *Official History of the Australian Army Medical Services 1914–1918.* Canberra: Australian War Memorial, 1930–1943.
Butler, J *Precarious Life: The Power of Mourning and Violence.* London: Verso, 2004.
Butler, J. "'Very Busy in Bosches Alley': One Day of the Somme in Sister Kit McNaughton's Diary." *Health & History* 6, no. 2 (2004): 18–32.
Carden-Coyne, A. *Reconstructing the Body: Classicism, Modernism, and the First World War.* Oxford: Oxford University Press, 2009.
Cartwright, L. *Screening the Body: Tracing Medicine's Visual Culture.* Minneapolis: University of Minnesota Press, 1995.
Chrastil, R. "The French Red Cross, War Readiness and Civil Society, 1866–1914." *French Historical Studies* 31, no. 3 (Summer 2008): 455–76.
Chrastil, R. *Organizing for War: France 1870–1914.* Baton Rouge: Louisiana State University Press, 2010.
Clampett, M. E. *My Dear Mother.* Melbourne: Muriel Clampett, 1992.
Clermont, C. *Souvenirs de Parisiennes en temps de guerre.* Paris: Berger-Levrault, 1918.
Cooperman, S. *World War I and the American Novel.* Baltimore: Johns Hopkins University Press, 1967.
Cottington, D. *Cubism in the Shadow of War: The Avant-Garde and Politics in Paris 1905–1914.* New Haven, CT: Yale University Press, 1988.
Crane, S. *The Red Badge of Courage.* Oxford: Oxford University Press, 1995 [1895].
Crémieux, J. *Croquis d'heures vécues, 1914–1919.* Fourmies: Imp. Bachy, 1934.
Curie, M., *La Radiologie et la guerre* (Paris: Fayard, 1921).
d'Alix, A. *La Croix-rouge française. Le rôle patriotique de femmes.* Paris: Perrin et cie., 1914.
Damousi, J. *The Labour of Loss: Mourning, Memory and Wartime Bereavement in Australia.* Melbourne: Cambridge University Press, 1999.

Damousi, J., and M. Lake, eds. *Gender and War: Australians at War in the Twentieth Century*. Cambridge: Cambridge University Press, 1995.

Darrow, M. H. "French Volunteer Nursing and the Myth of War Experience in World War I." *American Historical Review* 101, no. 1 (1996): 80–106.

Darrow, M. H. *French Women and the First World War: War Stories of the Home Front*. Oxford: Berg, 2000.

Darrow, M. H. "The Story of Franco-Prussian War Heroine Coralie Cahen and the French Red Cross, 1871–1914." *Proceedings of the Western Society for French History* 36 (2008): 167–80.

Das, S. "'The Impotence of Sympathy': Touch and Trauma in the Memoirs of First World War Nurses." *Textual Practice* 19, no. 2 (2005): 239–62.

Das, S. *Touch and Intimacy in First World War Literature*. Cambridge: Cambridge University Press, 2005.

Davies, C. *Gender and the Professional Predicament in Nursing*. Buckingham: Open University Press, 1995.

Dawson, G. *Soldier Heroes: British Adventure, Empire and the Imagining of Masculinities*. London: Routledge, 1994.

Deland, M. *Small Things*. New York: D. Appleton and Co., 1919.

Delmas, D. M. "Comment Soeur Julie sauva son hôpital et ses blessés." *La Croix des Landes* (20 December 1914).

de Man, P. *Blindness and Insight: Essays in the Rhetoric of Contemporary Criticism*. 2nd ed. Introduction by W. Godzich. London: Methuen, 1983.

Dent, O. *A VAD in France*. London: Grant Richards, 1917.

de Trailles, P., and H. de Trailles. *Les Femmes de France pendant la guerre et les deux sièges de Paris*. Paris: F. Polo Libraire-éditeur, 1872.

de Valdor, A. "Les Femmes décorées." *La Femme et la famille* 57, no. 8 (August 1889).

de Witt-Guizot, F. *La Femme et la guerre: Comment une femme peut-elle servir la France en temps de guerre?* Autun: Imprimerie Pernot, 1913.

d'Ezerville, Abbe F. J. *Nos bonnes religieuses françaises: leurs états de service dans les classes, dans les orphelinats, dans les hôpitaux, pendant la guerre de 1871, près des vieillards*. Paris: Pené Haton, librairie-éditeur, 1877.

Didierjean, B.-J. "Le Comte Henri de Verthamon, un héros de Loigny." *Etudes religieuses, philosophiques, historiques et littéraires, . . . publiées par des Pères de la Compagnie de Jésus,* 27, no. 51 (September–December 1890): 260–64.

Dietrick, J. "Seeing Battle, Knowing War: Feminist Re-Visioning in Hortensia Papadat-Bengescu's 'The Man Whose Heart They Could See.'" *Journal of International Women's Studies* 4, no. 3 (2003): 98–108.

Donnell, A. *Letters of an Australian Army Sister*. Sydney: Angus and Robertson, 1920.

Donoghue, D. *The American Classics: A Personal Essay*. New Haven, CT: Yale University Press, 2005.

Du Camp, M. *Paris bienfaisant*. Paris: Librairie Hachette, 1888.

Du Camp, M. "La Croix-rouge de France." Part 2, *Revue des deux mondes* 58, no. 90 (15 November 1888).

Duchaussoy, Dr. A. "Introduction," *L'Ecole des ambulancières et des garde-malades*. 4th ed. Paris: Association des Dames françaises, 1906.

Dugast, Dr. H. *Souvenirs intimes de l'ambulance mobile de la Côte d'Or: Campagnes de la Loire et de l'Est, 1870–1871*. Dijon: J. Marchand, 1871.

Durdin, J. *They Became Nurses: A History of Nursing in South Australia 1836–1980*. North Sydney, NSW: Allen and Unwin, 1991.

Eckstein, M. *Rites of Spring: The Great War and the Birth of the Modern Age*. Boston: Houghton Mifflin Company, 1989.

Emerson, R. Waldo. "The American Scholar" (1837), in *Collected Works*. 5 vols. Ed. R. E. Spiller and A. Ferguson, 52–70. Cambridge, MA: Harvard University Press, 1973.
Fell, A. S. "Myth, Countermyth and the Politics of Memory: Vera Brittain and Madeleine Clemenceau Jacquemaire's Interwar Nurse Memoirs." *Synergies* 4 (2011): 11–22.
Fell, A. S. "Nursing the Other: The Representation of Colonial Troops in French and British Nursing Memoirs," in *Race, Empire and First World War Writing*, ed. S. Das, 158–74. Cambridge: Cambridge University Press, 2011.
Ferenczi, S. *The Clinical Diary of Sandor Ferenczi*, ed. J. Dupont and N. Zarday Jackson. Cambridge, MA: Harvard University Press, 1988 [1932].
Finzi, K. *Eighteen Months in the War Zone: The Record of a Woman's Work on the Western Front*. London: Cassell and Company, 1916.
Fitzgerald, A. L. F. *The Edith Cavell nurse from Massachusetts A Record of One Year's Personal Service with the British Expeditionary Force in France, Boulogne: The Somme, 1916–1917, with an Account of the Imprisonment, Trial and Death of Edith Cavell*. Boston: W. A. Butterfield, 1917.
Fontanges, H. *La Légion d'honneur et les femmes décorées*. Paris: Alliance coopérative du livre, 1905.
Foucault, M. *The Birth of the Clinic: An Archaeology of Medical Perception*. Trans. A. M. Sheridan Smith. New York: Pantheon, 1973 [1963].
France, J. *Les Femmes françaises pendant la guerre, 1870*. Limoges: Marc Barbou et cie., 1887.
Fraser, H. *Women and War Work*. New York: G. Arnold Shaw, 1917.
Freedman, A. "Mary Borden's Forbidden Zone: Women's Writing from No-Man's Land." *Modernism/Modernity* 9, no. 1 (2002): 109–24.
Fussell, P. *The Great War and Modern Memory*. Oxford: Oxford University Press, 2000 [1975].
Gallagher, J. *The World Wars through the Female Gaze*. Carbondale: Southern Illinois University Press, 1998.
Gamarnikow, E. "Nurse or Woman: Gender and Professionalism in Reformed Nursing 1860–1923," in *Anthropology and Nursing*, ed. P. Holden and J. Littlewood, 110–29. London: Routledge, 1991.
Gammage, B. *The Broken Years: Australian Soldiers in the Great War*. Canberra: Penguin Books, 1975.
Garcia, H. Dicken, and G. Dell'Orto. *Hated Ideas and the American Civil War Press*. Spokane: Marquette Books, 2007.
Gibelli, A. *La Grande Guerra degli Italiani, 1915–1918*. Milan: Coen and Co., 1998.
Gill, J. "The Origins of the Australian Army Nursing Service and Its Involvement in the First World War." *ANU Historical Journal* 15 (1981/1987): 58–70.
Gleason, A. *Our Part in the Great War*. New York: Frederick A. Stokes Co., 1917.
Godfroy, L. *Souvenirs d'ambulance et de captivité (Noyon à Holzminden)*. Paris: L'Eclair, 1917.
Goldman, D. *Women Writers and the Great War*. New York: Twayne, 1995.
Goodman, P. *Women, Sexuality and War*. Houndmills: Palgrave Macmillan, 2002.
Goodman, R. *Our War Nurses: The History of the Royal Australian Army Nursing Corps, 1902–1988*. Brisbane: Boolarong Publications, 1988.
Gordon, A. Knyvett. "Some Thoughts on the War." *British Journal of Nursing* 53 (22 August 1914): 156–57.
Gould, J. "Women's Military Services in First World War Britain," in *Behind the Lines: Gender and the Two World Wars*, ed. M. Higonnet, J. Jenson, S. Michel and M. Collins Weitz, 114–25. New Haven, CT: Yale University Press, 1987.
Graves, R. *Goodbye to All That*. London: Jonathan Cape, 1929.

Grayzel, S. *Women's Identities at War: Gender, Motherhood, and Politics in Britain and France during the First World War.* Chapel Hill: University of North Carolina Press, 1999.
Grillet, M. "Un convoi de blessés (Janville 1870)." *La Revue du siècle, littéraire, artistique & scientifique* 3, no. 3 (1889): 1–3.
Gullace, N. *"The Blood of our Sons": Men, Women, and the Renegotiation of British Citizenship during the Great War.* Houndmills: Palgrave Macmillan, 2002.
Gurry, M. "Descent into the Other." *Age* (24 November 2001): 6.
Hallett, C. E. *Containing Trauma: Nursing Work in the First World War.* Manchester: Manchester University Press, 2009.
Hallett, C. E. "The Personal Writings of First World War Nurses: A Study of the Interplay of Authorial Intention and Scholarly Interpretation." *Nursing Inquiry* 14, no. 4 (2007): 320–29.
Hallett, C. E. "Portrayals of Suffering: Perceptions of Trauma in the Writings of First World War Nurses and Volunteers." *Canadian Bulletin of Medical History* 27, no. 1 (2011): 65–84.
Harouel, V. *Histoire de la Croix-Rouge.* Paris: Presses Universitaires de France, 1999.
Harris, B. *Blue and Gray in Black and White: Newspapers in the American Civil War.* Washington: Brassey's, 2000.
Harris, K. *More than Bombs and Bandages. Australian Army Nurses at Work in World War I.* Newport, NSW: Big Sky Publishing, 2010.
Hector, W. *Ethel Bedford Fenwick.* London: Royal College of Nursing, 1973.
Higonnet, M. "Authenticity and Art in Trauma Narratives of World War I." *Modernism/Modernity* 9, no. 1 (2002): 91–107.
Higonnet, M. *Lines of Fire. Women Writers of World War I.* Harmondsworth: Penguin, 1999.
Higonnet, M. *Nurses at the Front: Writing the Wounds of the Great War.* Boston: Northeastern University Press, 2001.
Higonnet, M. "X-Ray Vision: Women Photograph War." *Miranda* 2 (July 2010), available online at http://www.miranda-ejournal.eu/sdx2/miranda/index_numero.xsp?numero=2.
Higonnet, M., J. Jenson, S. Michel, and M. Collins Weitz, eds., *Behind the Lines: Gender and the Two World Wars.* New Haven, CT: Yale University Press, 1987.
Hogan G. F. *Experiences of a "Dinki Di" R.R.C. Nurse.* Sydney: Australasian Medical Publishing Company, 1933.
Hogenhuis-Seliverstoff, A. *Juliette Adam.* Paris: L'Harmattan, 2001.
Holder, V. L. "From Hand-Maiden to Right Hand: World War I—The Mud and the Blood." *AORN Journal* 80, no. 4 (2004): 652–65.
Holmes, K. "Day Mothers and Night Sisters: World War I Nurses and Sexuality," in *Gender and War: Australians at War in the Twentieth Century*, ed. J. Damousi and M. Lake, 43–59. Melbourne: Cambridge University Press, 1995.
Horne, P. "Henry James and 'The Forces of Violence': On the Track of 'Big Game' in 'The Jolly Corner'" *Henry James Review* 27, no. 3 (2006): 237–47.
Horne, P. "Reinstated: James in Roosevelt's Washington." *Cambridge Quarterly* 37, no. 1 (2008): 47–63.
Hunton, A. W., and K.M. Johnson. *Two Colored Women with the American Expeditionary Forces.* Brooklyn, NY: Brooklyn Eagle Press, 1920.
Hurcombe, M. "Raising the Dead: Visual Representations of the Combatant's Body in Interwar France." *Journal of War and Culture Studies* 1, no. 2 (2008): 159–74.
Hutchinson, J. F. *Champions of Charity: War and the Rise of the Red Cross.* Boulder, CO: Westview Press, 1996.

Inglis, E. "The Tragedy of Serbia." *Englishwoman* 30 (1916): 166.
Jablonski, L. *Les Femmes françaises à la guerre.* Paris Henri Charles-Lavanauzelle, 1894.
Jensen, K. *Mobilizing Minerva: American Women in the First World War.* Urbana: University of Illinois Press, 2008.
Johnson, K. *Henry James and the Visual.* Cambridge: Cambridge University Press, 2007.
Kaplan, L. "Deformities of the Great War: The Narratives of Mary Borden and Helen Zenna Smith." *Women and Language* 27, no. 2 (2004): 35–43.
Keegan, J. *The First World War.* London: Pimlico, 1999.
Kent, S. Kingsley. *Making Peace: The Reconstruction of Gender in Interwar Britain.* Princeton, NJ: Princeton University Press, 1993.
King, A. *Memorials of the Great War in Britain: The Symbolism and Politics of Remembrance.* Oxford: Berg, 1998.
Knibiehler, Y. *Cornettes et blouses blanches: Les infirmières dans la société française, 1880–1980.* Paris: Hachette, 1984.
Kramer, A. R. "Prisoners in the First World War," in *Prisoners in War,* ed. S. Scheipers, 75–90. Oxford: Oxford University Press, 2010.
Krippner, M. *The Quality of Mercy.* London: David and Charles, 1980.
Krob, M. Norman, "Commentary on 'Rosa.'" *Academic Medicine: The Journal of the Association of American Medical Colleges* 77, no. 7 (2002): 710–11.
Kuhlman, E. A. *Petticoats and White Feathers: Gender Conformity, Race, the Progressive Peace Movement, and the Debate Over War, 1895–1919.* Westport, CT: Praeger, 1997.
Lack, J. ed. *Anzac Remembered.* Melbourne: Department of History, University of Melbourne, 1998.
Laffin, J. *Damn the Dardanelles.* Sydney: Doubleday, 1980.
Lamberti, E., and V. Fortunati, eds. *Memories and Representations of War: The Case of World War I and World War II.* Amsterdam, Netherlands: Rodopi, 2009.
La Motte, E. N. *The Backwash of War: The Human Wreckage of the Battlefield as Witnessed by an American Hospital Nurse.* New York: G. P. Putnam's Sons, 1934 [1916].
Laqueur, T. W. "Memory and Naming in the Great War," in *Commemorations: The Politics of National Identity,* ed. J. R. Gillis, 150–66. Princeton, NJ: Princeton University Press, 1994.
Lee, J. "A Nurse and a Soldier: Gender, Class and National Identity in the First World War Adventures of Grace McDougall and Flora Sandes." *Women's History Review* 15, no. 1 (March 2006): 83–103.
Leed, E. J. *No Man's Land: Combat and Identity in World War I.* New York: Cambridge University Press, 1979.
Le Fort, Dr. L. *La Chirurgie militaire et les sociétés de secours en France et à l'étranger.* Paris: Librairie Germer Baillière, 1872.
Leighten, P. "Picasso's Collages and the Threat of War, 1912–13." *Art Bulletin* 67, no. 4 (1985): 653–72.
Leighten, P. *Re-Ordering the Universe: Picasso and Anarchism, 1897–1914.* Princeton, NJ: Princeton University Press, 1989.
Lejars, F. *Un Hôpital militaire à Paris pendant la guerre: Villemin 1914–1919.* Paris: Masson et cie., 1923.
Le Naour, J.-Y. *Misères et tourments de la chair durant la Grande Guerre.* Paris: Aubier, 2002.
Leneman, L. *In the Service of Life: The Story of Elsie Inglis and the Scottish Women's Hospitals.* Edinburgh: Mercat Press, 1994.

Leneman, L. "Medical Women at War 1914–1918." *Medical History* 38 (1994): 160–77.

Lentz-Smith, A. *Freedom Struggles: African Americans and World War I.* Cambridge, MA: Harvard University Press, 2009.

Léra, M. *Les Provinces françaises pendant la guerre.* Paris: Librairie académique, Perrin et cie., 1918.

Levée, M. "Faibles femmes . . . Femmes héroïques." *Minerva* (26 December 1937).

Lindenmeyr, A. *Poverty Is Not a Vice: Charity, Society and the State in Imperial Russia.* Princeton, NJ: Princeton University Press, 1996.

Luard, K. *Unknown Warriors.* London: Chatto and Windus, 1930.

Macdonald, L. *The Roses of No Man's Land.* London: Michael Joseph, 1980.

Macnaughtan, S. *A Woman's Diary of the War.* London: Thomas Nelson and Sons, 1915.

Malvern, S. "'For King and Country': Frampton's Edith Cavell (1915–1920) and the Writing of Gender in Memorials to the Great War," in *Sculpture and the Pursuit of a Modern Ideal in Britain, 1880–1930*, ed. D. Getsy, 219–44. Aldershot: Ashgate, 2004.

Mann, S., ed., *The War Diary of Clare Gass, 1915–1918.* Montreal: McGill Queen's University Press, 2000.

Marcus, J. "Corpus/Corps/Corpse: Writing the Body in/at War," in *Arms and the Woman: War, Gender and Literary Representation*, ed. H. M. Cooper, A. A. Munich, and S. M. Squier, 124–67. Chapel Hill: University of North Carolina Press, 1989.

Marquise de Foucault. *A Château at the Front.* Trans. G. B. Ives. Boston: Houghton Mifflin Company, 1931.

McEwen, Y. *"It's a Long Way to Tipperary" British and Irish Nurses in the Great War.* Dunfermline: Cualann Press, 2006.

McGann, S. *The Battle of the Nurses. A Study of Eight Women Who Influenced the Development of Professional Nursing, 1880–1930.* London: Scutari Press, 1992.

McPherson, K. "Carving Out a Past: The Canadian Nurses' Association War Memorial." *Histoire Sociale/Social History* 29 (1996): 417–29.

Millard, S. *I Saw Them Die: Diary and Recollections.* New York: Harcourt, Brace and Company, 1936.

Millicent, Duchess of Sutherland. *Six Weeks at the War.* London: The Times, 1914.

Mitchell, W. J. T. *Picture Theory.* Chicago: Chicago University Press, 1994.

Mitchell, D. *Women on the War Path: The Story of the Women of the First World War.* London: Cape, 1966.

Moore, J. *A Zeal for Responsibility.* Athens: University of Georgia Press, 1988.

Morgan, D. "Theatre of War: Combat, the Military, and Masculinities," in *Theorizing Masculinities*, ed. H. Brod and M. Kaufman, 165–82. Thousand Oaks, CA: Sage Publications, 1994.

Moriarty, C. "Private Grief and Public Remembrance: British First World War Memorials," in *War and Memory in the Twentieth Century*, ed. M. Evans and K. Lunn, 125–42. Oxford: Berg, 1997.

Mortimer, M. *A Green Tent in Flanders.* Garden City, NY: Doubleday, Page and Co., 1917.

Moynier, G. *La Croix-Rouge: son passé et son avenir.* Paris: Sandoz and Thuillier, 1882.

Mulvey, L. "Visual Pleasure and Narrative Cinema." *Screen* 16, no. 3 (1973): 6–18.

Nelson, S. "The Fork in the Road: Nursing History versus History of Nursing?" *Nursing History Review* 10 (2002): 175–88.
Noble, I. *Nurse around the World: Alice Fitzgerald*. New York: Messner, 1964.
Normand, J. "Association des Dames françaises: Madame Coralie Cahen." *La Revue bleue* 26, no. 2 (12 January 1889): 60.
Ouditt, S. *Fighting Forces, Writing Women: Identity and Ideology in the First World War*. London: Routledge, 1994.
Oxford, M. N. *Nursing in War Time: Lessons for the Inexperienced*. London: Methuen and Co., 1914.
Paget, Lady L. *With Our Serbian Allies: Second Report*. Printed for private circulation, 1916.
Parsons, R. Peabody. "Have We Kept the Faith?" *Atlantic Monthly* (August 1923): 666–72.
Petrović, I. "Foreign Medical Help in Serbian Liberation Wars from 1912 until 1918." *Arch Oncol* 18, no. 4 (2010): 143–48.
Pickles, K. *Transnational Outrage: The Death and Commemoration of Edith Cavell*. Basingstoke: Palgrave, 2005.
Piédagnel. *Les Ambulances de Paris pendant le siège (1870–1871)*. Paris: Librairie générale, 1871.
Poole, Sister A. "The Trivial Round." *Australasian Nurses Journal* 14, no. 11 (15 November 1916).
Potter, J. *Boys in Khaki, Girls in Print: Women's Literary Responses to the Great War 1914–1918*. Oxford: Oxford University Press, 2005.
Pratt, R. "Nursing at Lemnos—August—December, 1915." *Reveille* 6, no. 12 (1 August 1933): 42.
Prior R. M., and W. S. Marble. "The Overlooked Heroines: Three Silver Star Nurses of World War I." *Military Medicine* 173, no. 5 (2008): 493–98.
Rae, R. *Scarlet Poppies: The Army Experience of Australian Nurses during World War One*. Burwood, NSW: College of Nursing, 2004.
Rae, R. *Veiled Lives. Threading Australian Nursing History into the Fabric of the First World War*. Burwood, NSW: College of Nursing, 2009.
Rathbone, I. *We That Were Young*. London: Virago Press, 1988 [1932].
Rees, P. *The Other Anzacs*. Sydney: Allen and Unwin, 2008.
Richard, J. "Un convoi de blessés (Janville 1870)." *La Revue du siècle, littéraire, artistique & scientifique* 3, no. 3 (1889): 4–5.
Robson, L. "The Origins and Character of the First AIF, 1914–1918: Some Statistical Evidence." *Historical Studies* 15, no. 61 (October 1973): 737–49.
Roetter, C. *The Art of Psychological Warfare, 1914–1945*. New York: Stein and Day, 1974.
Ruault, L. *Cent ans de Croix-Rouge Française au service de l'humanité*. Paris: Hachette, 1964.
Ryder, M. R. "'Dear, Tender-Hearted, Uncomprehending America': Dorothy Canfield Fisher's and Edith Wharton's Fictional Responses to the First World War," in *The Literature of the Great War Reconsidered: Beyond Modern Memory*, ed. P.J. Quinn and S. Trout, 143–55. Basingstoke: Palgrave, 2001.
Said, E. W. *Orientalism*. London: Penguin, 2003.
Sarnecky, M. *A History of the US Army Nurse Corps*. Philadelphia: University of Pennsylvania Press, 1999.
Sassoon, S. *Complete Memoirs of George Sherston*. London: Faber and Faber, 1937.
Sassoon, S. *Memoirs of an Infantry Officer*. London: Faber and Faber, 2000 [1930].
Scardino Belzer, A. "The Other Army: Italian Women on the Home Front During the First World War." *Minerva Journal of Women and War* 3, no. 1 (2009): 6–23.

Scarry, E. *The Body in Pain: The Making and Unmaking of the World*. Oxford: Oxford University Press, 1985.
Scates, B., and R. Frances. *Women and the Great War*. Melbourne: Cambridge University Press, 1997.
Schultheiss, K. *Bodies and Souls: Politics and the Professionalization of Nursing in France, 1880–1922*. Cambridge, MA: Harvard University Press, 2001.
Shaw McLaren, E. *A History of the Scottish Women's Hospitals*. London: Hodder and Stoughton, 1919.
Sherman, D. *The Construction of Memory in Interwar France*. Chicago: University of Chicago Press, 1999.
Smith, A. K. *The Second Battlefield: Women, Modernism and the First World War*. Manchester: Manchester University Press, 2000.
Smith, A. K. "The Woman Who Dared: Major Mabel St. Clair Stobart," in *The Women's Movement in Wartime: International Perspectives 1914–19*, ed. A. S. Fell and I. Sharp, 158–74. Basingstoke: Palgrave, 2007.
Smith, A. K. *Women's Writing of the First World War: An Anthology*. Manchester: Manchester University Press, 2000.
Smith, L. *Four Years out of Life*. Glasgow: Philip Allan, 1931.
Sniter, C. "La gloire des femmes célèbres: Métamorphoses et disparité de la statuaire publique parisienne de 1870 à nos jours." *Sociétés et Représentations* 26 (2008): 153–70.
Squires, A., ed. *One Hundred Percent American*. New York: George H. Doran, 1918.
Stein, G. *Wars I Have Seen*. London: Brilliance Books, 1984 [1945].
Stimson, J. "The Army Nurse Corps," in *The Medical Department of the United States Army in the World War*. Vol. XIII, Part Two, 287–354. Washington, DC: US Government Printing Office, 1927.
Stimson, J. *Finding Themselves: The Letters of an American Army Chief Nurse in a British Hospital in France* . New York: Macmillan, 1918.
Stobart, St Clair, "Women's Work in War." *British Journal of Nursing* 53 (18 July 1914): 53.
Strachan, H. *The First World War*. London: Simon and Schuster, 2003.
Strachey, R. *The Cause*. London: Virago, 1978 [1928].
Summers, A. *Angels and Citizens: British Women as Military Nurses, 1854–1914*. Rev. ed. Newbury: Berks, Threshold Press, 2000.
Taithe, B. *Defeated Flesh: Welfare, Warfare and the Making of Modern France*. Manchester: Manchester University Press, 1999.
Tate, T. *Modernism, History, and the First World War*. Manchester: Manchester University Press, 1998.
Thébaud, F. *La Femme au temps de la guerre de 14*. Paris: Editions Stock, 1986.
Thébaud, F. "La Grande Guerre," in *Histoire des femmes en occident 5: Le XXe siècle*, ed. G. Duby, 31–74. Paris: Plon, 1992.
Thom, D. *Nice Girls and Rude Girls: Women Workers in World War I*. London: I. B. Tauris, 1998.
Thomson, A. *Anzac Memories: Living with the Legend*. Oxford: Oxford University Press, 1995.
Thurstan, V. *A Text Book of War Nursing*. London: G. P. Putnam's Sons, 1917.
Thwing, C. F. *The American Colleges & Universities in the Great War, 1914–1919: A History*. New York: Macmillan, 1920.
Tilton, M. *The Grey Battalion*. Sydney: Angus and Robertson, 1934 [1933].
Tison, S. "Traumatisme de guerre et commémorations: Comment Champenois et Sarthois sont-ils sortis de la guerre? (1870–1940)." *Guerres mondiales et conflits contemporains* 216 (October 2004): 5–29.

Todman, D. *The Great War: Myth and Memory.* London: Hambledon Continuum, 2005.

Tomida, H., and G. Daniels, eds. *Japanese Women Emerging from Subservience.* Folkestone: Global Oriental, 2005.

Turquan, J. *1870–1871: Les femmes de France pendant l'invasion.* Paris: Berger-Levrault et cie., 1893.

Tylee, C. M. *The Great War and Women's Consciousness: Images of Militarism and Womanhood in Women's Writings, 1914–1964.* Houndmills: Macmillan, 1990.

Tylee, C. M. "The Spectacle of War: Photographs of the Russian Front by Florence Farmborough." *Women: A Cultural Review* 8, no. 1 (1997): 65–80.

van Bergen, L. *Before My Helpless Sight: Suffering, Dying and Military Medicine on the Western Front, 1914–1918.* Farnham, Surrey: Ashgate, 2009.

van Vorst, M. *War Letters of an American Woman.* New York: John Lane Co., 1916.

Van Weinen, M. *Partisans and Poets: The Political Work of American Poetry in the Great War.* Cambridge: Cambridge University Press, 1997.

Watson, J. S. K. *Fighting Different Wars: Experience, Memory and the First World War in Britain.* Cambridge: Cambridge University Press, 2004.

Watson, J. S. K. "Khaki Girls, VADs, and Tommy's Sisters: Gender and Class in First World War Britain." *International History Review* 13, no. 1 (1997): 32–51.

Watson, J. S. K. "Wars in the Wards: The Social Construction of Medical Work in First World War Britain." *Journal of British Studies* 41 (2002): 484–510.

Wharton, E. *Fighting France from Dunkerque to Belfort.* New York: Charles Scribner's Sons, 1919.

Whitman, W. *Leaves of Grass.* Ed. S. Bradley. New York: Norton, 1973.

Winter, J. *Sites of Memory, Sites of Mourning: The Great War in European Cultural History.* Cambridge: Cambridge University Press, 1995.

Woolf, V. *A Room of One's Own.* New York: Harcourt Brace, 1929.

Woollacott, A. "'Khaki Fever' and Its Control: Gender, Class, Age and Sexual Morality on the British Homefront in the First World War." *Journal of Contemporary History* 29, no. 2 (1994): 325–47.

Young, M., ed. *"We Are Here, Too."* Adelaide: Australian Down Syndrome Association Incorporated, 1991.

Zeiger, S. *In Uncle Sam's Service: Women Workers with the American Expeditionary Force, 1917–1919.* Ithaca, NY: Cornell University Press, 1999.

Contributors

Carol Acton is Associate Professor of English at Saint Jerome's University in the University of Waterloo. Her book, *Grief in Wartime: Private Pain, Public Discourse* (Palgrave Macmillan, 2007), includes discussion of First World War nurses. She has also published articles and book chapters on medical personnel, gender, and war in the twentieth century. Her current project, with Dr. Jane Potter, is on trauma and resilience in medical personnel working in war zones.

Margaret H. Darrow earned her PhD in History from Rutgers University; she has been on the faculty of Dartmouth College in New Hampshire since 1980. A specialist in modern French history, she teaches courses about the French Revolution, industrialization, and the First World War. She is the author of *Revolution in the House: Family, Class and Inheritance in Southern France, 1775–1825* (Princeton University Press, 1989) and *French Women and the First World War: War Stories of the Home Front* (Berg Publishers, 2000). Her current research concerns women's patriotic mobilization prior to the First World War.

Alison S. Fell is Professor of French Cultural History at the University of Leeds. She has published widely on French and British women and the First World War, including two edited volumes: (with Ingrid Sharp) *The Women's Movement in Wartime: International Perspectives 1914–1919* (Palgrave Macmillan, 2007) and *Les Femmes face à la guerre* (Peter Lang, 2009). She is currently completing a monograph, *Back to the Front: Women as Veterans in France and Britain, 1916–33*, and is leading an AHRC-funded research project entitled "Legacies of War 1914–18/2014–18."

Christine E. Hallett is Professor of Nursing History at the University of Manchester, UK. She is chair of the UK Association for the History of Nursing and was founding chair of the European Association for the History of Nursing. Professor Hallett holds Fellowships of the Royal Society of Medicine, UK, and the Royal Society for the Arts, UK. Her publications include the critically acclaimed monograph *Containing Trauma: Nursing Work in the First World War* (Manchester University Press, 2009) and the popular *Celebrating Nurses: A Visual History* (Fil Rouge Press, 2010).

Kirsty Harris completed her PhD on the work of Australian Army nurses in World War I at the University of Melbourne in 2007, and received the C.E.W. Bean Prize for Military History in 2008. She is currently an honorary fellow at the University of Melbourne and has published a number of articles on military nursing work including on nurse anesthetists, nursing at sea, British–Australian nursing relationships during World War I, and postwar nursing work. Her first book is entitled *More than Bombs and Bandages: Australian Army Nurses at Work in World War I* (Regimental Books, 2011).

Margaret R. Higonnet is Professor of English and Comparative Literature at the University of Connecticut and an affiliate at the Center for European Studies, Harvard University. A past president of the American Conference on Romanticism and of the American Comparative Literature Association, her interests range from romantic literary theories to children's literature, Thomas Hardy, and comparative feminist criticism (see *Borderwork* (Cornell University Press, 1994), and *Comparatively Queer* (Palgrave, 2010)). Much of her scholarship has been devoted to the literature of World War I, as in *Behind the Lines* (Yale University Press, 1987), *Lines of Fire* (Penguin/Plume, 1999), and *Nurses at the Front* (Northeastern University Press, 2001).

Hazel Hutchison teaches English Literature at the University of Aberdeen. She researches British and American literature of the late nineteenth century and the early twentieth century, and has written books and articles about Henry James, Gerard Manley Hopkins, and Rupert Brook. She has edited Mary Borden's war text *The Forbidden Zone* (Hesperus, 2008), and she is currently writing a book about American literature of the First World War.

Jane Potter is Senior Lecturer in Publishing at the Oxford International Centre for Publishing Studies, Oxford Brookes University. Her publications include *Boys in Khaki, Girls in Print: Women's Literary Responses to the Great War 1914–1918* (Oxford University Press, 2005), an edition of the First World War novel *Good Old Anna* by Marie Belloc Lowndes (Pickering and Chatto, 2010), and *Three Poets of the First World War: Ivor Gurney, Isaac Rosenberg and Wilfred Owen*, with Jon Stallworthy (Penguin, 2011). Her work with Carol Acton, "'These Frightful Sights Would Work Havoc with One's Brain': Subjective Experience, Trauma and Resilience in the Narratives of Medical Personnel in the First World

War," is published in *Literature and Medicine* 30, no. 1 (Spring 2012). She is editor of the *Wilfred Owen Association Journal.*

Angela K. Smith is a Reader in English at Plymouth University. She is the author of a number of books and articles on women and the First World War, including: *Suffrage Discourse in Britain During the First World War* (Ashgate, 2005); ed., *Gender and Warfare in the Twentieth Century: Textual Representations* (Manchester University Press, 2004); ed., *Women's Writing of the First World War: An Anthology* (Manchester University Press, 2000); *The Second Battlefield: Women, Modernism and the First World War* (Manchester University Press, 2000). She was general editor for the five volume collection *British Literature of World War One* (Pickering and Chatto, 2011). As well as currently working on a monograph about the work and writings of British women in Serbia and Russia during the First World War, she is also co-editing a collection of essays: *War and Displacement.*

Janet S. K. Watson is the author of *Fighting Different Wars: Experience, Memory, and the First World War in Britain* (Cambridge University Press, 2004) which was awarded the Tomlinson Prize of the Western Front Association for the best history of the First World War in 2005. On the faculty of the Department of History at the University of Connecticut, Watson is currently working on several projects centering on commemorations of the anniversaries of key events of the Second World War and how they related to changing ideas about late twentieth-century British society.

Index